A GENTLE DEATH:
Personal Caregiving to the Terminally Ill

by

Elizabeth S. Callari, R.N.

Tudor Publishers, Inc.

A GENTLE DEATH:
Personal Caregiving to the Terminally Ill

First printing, June 1986
Second printing, January 1987
Third printing, March 1989

"Reflections of a Patient", by Patricia M. Ismert and Caroline M. Arnold, first appeared in the March 1978 issue of *Supervisor Nurse*. Used by permission.

Library of Congress Cataloging in Publication Data

Callari, Elizabeth S., 1935—

A gentle death.

1. Terminal care   2. Death.   3. Bereavement.
I. Title
R726.8.C35   1986   616'.029   85–31814
ISBN 0-936389-00-1
ISBN 0-936389-01-X (pbk.)

Printed in the United States of America

PUBLISHER'S NOTE

The information contained in this book is in no way intended to replace the advice, care, and counsel of a liscensed physician. Diagnosis and treatment of any illness should only be carried out by trained medical professionals. The views and opinions expressed herein are not necessarily those of the publisher.

This book is dedicated to the Golden Age of Enlightenment, and especially to all my teachers—those who have helped me along this path; my family, my friends, Ed, Bill, Elisabeth, Ram Dass, Warren, and to everyone I have ever met who has touched my life, even for a moment.

NAMASTE!

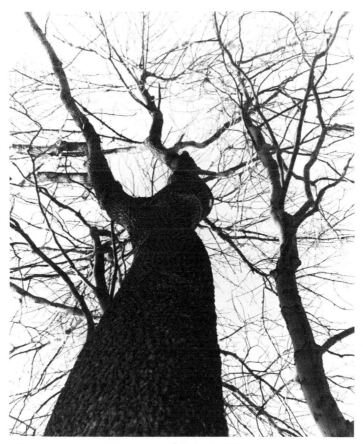

Photographs: Deborah Callari Myers

Table of Contents

Introduction

At age 50, I've come to divide my past life into two parts: the first part, when I feared death, and the second, when I didn't. Like most people, I've had other important life experiences, such as a long marriage, two wonderful children, a challenging career, a divorce, and so on. Like others, I've achieved a good deal, endured a good deal, and learned a lot. But for me, making sense of my life has depended on my confronting and understanding death.

I'm a registered nurse specializing in chemotherapy and in the counseling of terminally ill patients. All my adult life I've worked with ill people, yet only part of that time did I realize what was occuring right before my eyes when a person died. At first, I did everything I could to avoid, deny,overlook, or outrun the reality I saw in my work: that people die.

It wasn't easy to move from fearing death to being comfortable with it. Circumstances combined to force me to confront death, and I was very reluctant to participate in the drama. Afterwards, however, I realized that I had begun to walk this path as a child, and that I would continue to walk it.

Now, in the second part of my life, I walk joyfully. As I understand death, I more fully understand life. Several hundred people have shared their deaths with me. Each has helped teach and prepare me, and it is now my hope to help and prepare others: those who are dying, those who care for them, and all who love enough to peer deeply into the final experience of life.

Some years ago I began to have excessively heavy menstrual periods. Pap smears were inconclusive, but my inner self told me something was wrong. My regular gynecologist seemed unconcerned, so I searched until I found a physican more willing to listen. The night after my first visit to the new doctor, I had a remarkably clear dream in which I realized that I must have an operation.

My new doctor soon responded to my concern with his own. Surgery was performed.

Shortly after the operation, I watched a televised panel discussion from my hospital bed, a discussion on working with the dying, sponsored by the American Cancer Society. Ironically, I had been scheduled to participate on that panel.

But now I was watching it from the other side—as a possible cancer patient. Two days later, I woke up crying, and kept crying for several hours.

During that time, a nurse I knew came into my room. "Why are you crying?" she asked. "We're not used to seeing you this way."

Another nurse said, "Oh, I see you're not feeling well today. A bit blue, maybe?"

Why, indeed, did I cry? I was quite naturally very fearful about the possible diagnosis and didn't care about being a "good" patient. I felt terrible. "A bit blue" didn't begin to describe my feelings.

Early the next morning my doctor drew the curtains around the bed and grasped my hand. He told me I had cancer.

My mouth went dry, and I felt as if I were floating. *Leiomyosarcoma*, he said. *Encased in a fibroid tumor.* He asked me not to go to the library to read up on the prognosis. I agreed, and he left.

After the doctor was gone, I stepped to the bathroom mirror. The face I saw there did not seem to be mine—I was like a stranger to myself. Anger took hold, and my trembling became a series of long, racking shudders. I clutched the bathroom handrail, struggling for breath. More than anything else, I wanted to run down the hall shrieking with rage. But if I did, the staff surely would call for a psychiatric consultation. I could almost hear the nurses cluck, "My, my, you're not dealing with this very well, are you?" After all, I worked with the dying every day, didn't I? Wasn't I supposed to be the calm, all-knowing expert? But only the realization that my troubles would be compounded by hysterics kept me in the room.

It was, however, a long road that had led me to that hospital bed, and to a confrontation with my own fear and ignorance of death. Although I was an experienced nurse, much of my life had been spent avoiding or skirting the fact of death. I had been, like most other people, all too willing to avoid or evade the subject in my own mind, even though I worked with chronically or terminally ill patients every day.

All my life I wanted to be a nurse. As a little girl, I folded endless sheets of white paper and taped them just so to make myself little nurse's caps. As I crayoned bright red crosses on those little hats and balanced them properly on my head, I imagined myself all grown up, smiling and moving from one hospital bed to another, giving care and warmth and hope to my patients. Those patients, in turn, smiled gratefully up at me. They took their medication cheerfully, ate their meals, followed the doctor's orders, and finally got up and walked out of the hospital. They became whole again because of my tender care. Each and every one was restored to good health. Because of me.

This vision sustained me through nursing school. I was a very good nursing student, although rather lackadaisical in other subjects. I progressed rapidly toward my own real nurse's cap.

In every nursing class, the spoken or unspoken watchword was: "Don't become emotionally involved with your patients. Don't."

"How sad," I thought, but studied right along in a happy rush. I didn't bother to think about the real implications of that statement. My studies were too interesting. The six weeks I spent studying labor and delivery were thrilling, and I decided to specialize in obstetrical nursing: new life; glowing happy mothers; dramatic deliveries. That's what I wanted.

If our class spent six weeks learning about labor and delivery, we may have spent six minutes discussing death. In fact, I do not now remember a word being said in my nursing classes about patients dying. I knew people died, of course. I was dating an intern who soon started a residency in Pathology. He performed post-mortems as part of his training, and when our social plans were occasionally changed by an emergency autopsy, I would go along and help. It was, however, an exercise in weighing, measuring and observing organs, not a close-up look at death. The bodies were draped, the faces covered. These objects had nothing to do with me.

I fell in love with this doctor and we were married after my graduation. My husband took a position in Richmond, Virginia. I applied at the same hospital for work as an obstetrical nurse. However, the only position open was on the medical and surgical floor. I took it, hoping that a better position would open in the future.

One day when I came to work, another nurse said to me, "The patient in 4B expired."

Expired. An unemotional word. The patient had expired as a parking permit, a contract, or a driver's license would expire. But I felt frightened nonetheless.

The man who had died was not someone I had been assigned to care for, but I felt compelled to look into his room. I returned to the nursing station deeply shaken. I unrealistically felt, deep inside, that I could prevent this sort of thing from happening again by working harder and with more diligence than before.

The supervising nurse was a strong Mennonite woman, thin and reserved. She made no errors in giving medications and never, ever "got involved" with her patients. I tried very hard to model my behavior after her, but fell far short. I felt hopeless and completely lost when one of my patients died.

One patient was a young family man with leukemia. In those days, little could be done for him medically. I did not fully realize how very ill he was, and the fact that he might die—expire—was never mentioned. I had neither the experience nor the knowledge to contradict my belief that he would be getting well soon. His wife became more and more worried and upset, but for eight hours a day, I was in charge of his complete care, and I believed he would live. Wonderful young men with bright futures, loving wives, and everything to look forward to just didn't die.

He died.

I cried in grief and anger against the unfairness of the young man's death.

Soon, however, my feelings and questions were shut away as a new part of my life began. I became pregnant, withdrew from nursing, and left the frightening experiences behind. For the next fifteen years I evaded Death the failure, Death the terrifier. Life was good and full. Two children, a husband, a lovely home, and a fine social life were all mine.

Yet I was not free of my fear of the end of life.

Some years before my father died, he tried to prepare me for his eventual death. He owned several beautiful oil paintings and had placed my name on the back of one he particularly wanted me to inherit. When he showed this to me, obviously wanting to discuss it, I rejected the whole idea and ran from the room crying, "Don't you *ever* talk to me about dying. You and Mom just can't do that to me!"

That was an extreme reaction, but indicative of my deep-rooted fear and dread. The pattern had begun when I was a child. I don't remember anyone talking to me about death. But then, I didn't ask, either, because I was instinctively afraid of the answers. Death was, in some ways, a forbidden topic like sex, except that my mother could verify what my girlfriends had whispered to me on that subject.

Only in Sunday School was I taught something about death. "When you die, you go to heaven or hell," depending on how 'good' or 'bad' you had been during your lifetime. "Pray...Talk to God...ask him for what you want," I was taught. It was not suggested to me to *listen* to God, nor to trust that He surely knows what I need. Not until much later did I learn to listen and trust, and to stop resisting what *was.*

So, it seemed that I was protected during those years from the pain of death. The protection was illusory. I slowly began to learn that what I pushed away from myself would come back to me in one form or another. During a short span, three events occurred which I would not accept, but which I also could not control.

My greatly-loved father died suddenly while in Europe on a business trip. Then my husband and I separated and divorced. This also was a "death," the only difference being that my husband's physical presence was still visible to me. The third event was the death of my sixth-month-old nephew, Jeffrey. I remember very clearly my sister and her husband kneeling alongside the small white casket, pinning a pair of wings on Jeffrey's sleeping garment. The wings, I realized later, were symbolic of his freedom from the physical body. At that time, however, all I could feel was my own pain and rage at the injustice of his death.

The emotional impact of these events forced me to try to restructure my life. After beginning to evaluate the directions in which I could go, I met a man who I believe was sent to me for a very special reason, but for only a short time. He helped me piece my life back together and, more importantly, to learn how to love myself. But then he died, after giving me the gift of self-worth and self-love.

As a single person, I needed to provide for myself financially. I took a position as a labor and delivery nurse in a large city hospital. Surely, I thought, death would be less threatening in this environment. After working several months and experiencing the excitement and joy of birthing, I was faced with the birth of a stillborn child. The limp, bluish body, lacking any life-force, was promptly removed to a utility room and wrapped in a plastic shroud. A discussion among the nurses followed as to whether to baptize the remains.

One finally waved her hand over the infant's head and said quickly, "I baptize you in the name of the Father, Son and Holy Ghost. Amen."

In the recovery room the mother began asking to see her dead child—the remains of the life she had carried within her for almost nine months. The doctor immediately answered that it would not be in her best interests. It was not, he said, a good idea. The mother totally withdrew into herself and did not communicate with the staff for the duration of her stay in the hospital.

I was struck with the realization that, had this been my experience, I would have insisted on seeing for myself that my child had indeed been born dead.

Were doctors and nurses afraid of death? Was I also afraid? For the first time I honestly asked myself these questions, and answered yes, and again *yes*. My fear constricted my ability to live fully; my colleagues' fear, expressed in the behavior and attitudes accepted in the hospital, had reinforced my fear, just as they had damaged that mother with the stillborn child. I saw a chance to begin working on myself, on my relationship with death. I went into the utility room and unwrapped the tiny body. I held it, wept, and spoke aloud some of my feelings. It was as if a stone were lifted from my chest. A sense of lightness and relief came to me. Finally, I felt peace.

This was the real beginning of my spiritual and professional journey, a journey which, as I lay in my hospital bed after the diagnosis of cancer, had taken a sudden and frightening detour.

The best medical opinion gave me a year to live. For whatever reasons, I chose not to believe it. I began a "self-healing" program using imagery, music, and a positive attitude. I learned to truly listen to my body and follow its dictates. Again, for whatever reasons, healing was complete: I have now been asymptomatic for eight years.

My experience with cancer changed my life. My physician later said, "Elizabeth, I can't help but think you were destined to go through this, to find out what it's really like to know you have a serious illness." I believe he was absolutely right, for I have developed ideas and beliefs as a direct result of my experience and put those concepts to work for others.

Chapter One

The Caregiver

By some standards I'm considered a lousy counselor. When I'm working with the dying, I don't do a lot of things a counselor or therapist is expected to do. For instance, I don't use labels like "depressed, angry, denying, bargaining or accepting" to describe the dying person. Words like these, originally intended to denote very general categories of behavior, are sometimes used to identify the whole person. We hear, "He's in a depression" or "She is angry."

The therapist who wields the power of the profession against a vulnerable person creates an expectation of how that person will behave. The patient might inadvertently receive the message from the therapist: "You're depressed and angry now, and my specialized knowledge tells me that you'll stay that way." What choice has the patient, but to remain hostile and uncooperative? If this learned and powerful person says, "the patient's depressed," the patient thinks, "Then for sure I must be depressed!" So further depression is the result of the burden the dying person must bear.

I don't limit the feelings and expressions of the ones

I work with by applying labels to them. It is not my place to decide how they'll behave.

Another thing I don't do as a counselor is keep a "professional" distance between the dying person and myself. Some professional therapists keep a desk between themselves and the person with whom they are working. A broad, flat field of authority, the desk is often full of symbols of the therapist's importance. Papers, closed files, books with long titles, and diplomas may intimidate the patient.

As the dying person talks, the therapist writes— what? Somehow the dying person's words—and the ideas, feelings, and expressions that they represent— have become the private property of the therapist/ counselor, to perhaps be used in ways the original owner does not know. I find it most comfortable just sitting in a recliner next to the patient, close enough so that I can take a hand when the sharing becomes difficult. If I need to write down something about my work with that person, I wait for a private moment to do so, because pencil and paper can get in the way of communication.

Professional therapists usually dress differently than their patients, too. Crisp white coats or three- piece suits and ties present an imposing image to someone attired in a faded green hospital gown with the string ties missing. Symbolic vulnerability loses its abstract quality when the stylishly-garbed thera- pist meets the hospital-clad dying person. To avoid this contrast and "distance," I dress quite casually. My clothes are simple, colorful and comfortable, and serve as a reminder that the dying person and I share far more similarities than differences.

What I do as a counselor for the dying is to give love. Without conditions. Unwavering. I pull up a chair and cradle the dying friend in my arms, if necessary. I hug when hugging is wanted, or massage a weary body that is experiencing "skin hunger." I listen and laugh and cry—or stay silent. I offer to share my lunch, or to bring in a pizza. I run errands or carry messages.

Most Importantly, however, I open my heart and learn from the dying. "Degreed" counselors/therapists generally learn from books and school and each other; their patients may be sources of information, but not of real knowledge. I leave my intellect outside the door and put my arms around the person I'm working with and say, "I've never died before, so I can't imagine how you must be feeling. I'd like to become more comfortable with death myself, and I need your help to do this. Please share with me."

How the doors open! The dying are often our greatest teachers: short on time but long on the will to share the meaning of their lives, the dying speak straight from the heart. There is no time to be phony, no need to worry about what others might think. The dying person expects the same honesty and directness in return. And I believe they deserve it.

In my work with the dying, I open my heart and leave analysis behind. I seek oneness with the person, not fulfillment of a particular role or maintenance of a title. Simply to share, to help and to be helped, is my goal.

How can an ordinary person help one who is faced with serious illness and quite possibly death? People often express amazement upon learning about my work, and blurt out comments like, "How upsetting that must be! How do you manage?"

I was once introduced prior to a television documentary on our hospice as, "Elizabeth Callari, who by rights should be the most depressed person in Pinellas County. But she's not!" It was as if I had accomplished a small miracle in maintaining my usual cheerful countenance. This is an incorrect assumption, for working with the dying as a caregiver is wonderfully enriching.

The importance of this work lies in the fact that the depression, worry and anxiety which accompany a terminal illness are often more debilitating than the illness itself. Dying is not just physical; it happens to the whole person. We reckon with the social, emotional and spiritual aspects as well. In dying, as in living, the whole person requires recognition, response and care.

Every dying person needs to be surrounded by loved ones. And this work need not be done—in fact, it is best not done—by some sort of specialist. In my experience, the most successful caregivers and counselors for the dying have been good, ordinary people who understand the profound truth that neither they nor anyone else can plant corn and then harvest tomatoes. That is, fury does not bring calm, nor resentment, cooperation; fear cannot command knowledge, and contempt does not lead to love. To work with the dying is to step into an emotional field where these dichotomies and others must be felt, for they often defy logic. Advanced levels of education and training emphasize analysis and logic, which is the last thing dying people need.

Instead those facing death need the love and respect which affirm human worth and dignity. Caregivers, in a variety of relationships with the dying, can serve this fundamental need.

While I've worked with many caregivers who have given incredible service, two particularly come to mind now. One was a mother caring for her cancer-stricken adult son. Mrs. Josslin, who bordered on frailty herself, found the physical strength to care for Peter's every need for over ten hours each day. She struggled powerfully against her own wishes and hopes in order to help Peter toward a peaceful death, supporting her son's decisions about treatment which she, the mother, might have made differently. Mrs. Josslin made deviled eggs, Peter's favorite food, every day of the illness.

She boiled the eggs daily and mixed the yolks with diced pickles and mayonnaise, and put in the other spices Peter liked. Peter ate deviled eggs until the day he slipped tranquilly to his death, satisfied in the tangible evidence of his mother's understanding of his need to leave this world.

Like Mrs. Josslin, Lila persevered in her work as a caregiver and hospice volunteer. She worked with Dana, who lived with her two children as a family with Tom, a career soldier. Dana's son had become alienated from Tom and was placed in a foster home over his mother's helpless protests. The family was divided by animosity and distrust, but Lila was able to tread both gently and firmly among family members as her heart dictated. She listened to her inner feelings while her head told her she could not repair the situation. Lila was constantly afraid of making things worse for Dana. But the result of her work was, finally, a reunion—perhaps an imperfect one—but one which could not have happened at all without Lila's efforts.

Both these women planted the crops they most deeply wanted to reap: love, courage, and forgiveness. Mrs. Josslin and Peter achieved a caring closeness which had not been freely expressed during their prior busy lives. Lila, too, concentrated on love and calm within the storm; her determination was sorely tested by the pain of the family with which she worked. More than once these women doubted their abilities to persevere, but each faithfully tended their crops. And at last the harvest from the seeds of love, courage and forgiveness were bountiful.

Those who work with the dying need to learn to use another important quality: the ability to be nonjudgemental, to resist imposing one's own categories of "good" and "bad" onto another's experience. When I conduct educational seminars and workshops on the subject of death and dying, the book *Gramp* by Mark and Dan Jury is frequently mentioned by participants. Gramp's family allowed him to make his own decisions during his terminal illness, even to the point of refusing food and thus seemingly "starving" himself. People's reactions vary, of course, but when I hear people say, "How terrible, that family *let* Gramp lie without sheets on the bed," or "They *let* him wear his wife's nightgown," or "They *let* him lie without food or water!" then I know that part of my work must be to guide participants to understand that dying—the final earthly experience—is neither "good" nor "bad". It is, instead, an unchanging fact.

How death comes to each person is unique, an intimate process fully known only to that person. There is no set of experiences a dying person "should" have, and no guaranteed set of rules for caregivers and families. To point to components of a particular death and label some "good" and some "bad" slams the door to deeper understanding and spiritual closeness.

Letting go of prejudices, judgemental attitudes, and prior assumptions is a critical aspect of coming to terms with death and dying. A caregiver cannot achieve the fullest potential in helping the dying without completing this task. Filling each resulting vacancy in the heart with unconditional and unwavering love and respect for the dying is the key to tremendous growth, for the dying have a good deal to give to those of us who have not yet traveled so far on life's paths. Peter Josslin, for instance, taught me some important lessons.

When, as a hospice volunteer, I first met Peter, I was struck once more by the fragility of life. Lying in a bed framed by an ornately-carved Mediterranean-style headboard, Peter seemed fragile in his lime-green cotton gown. His hair stood sparse and perpendicular to his scalp,like an infant, and his chocolate-colored eyes seemed even darker against the paleness of his skin. The equipment he needed—oxygen tanks, a bedpan, the suction machine, an array of medications—ringed the bed.

As I sat beside Peter, getting acquainted, he let me know right away that his remaining days were very special and he didn't care for idle chatter. His time and energy were so limited and precious that he resented those who drained him with their pity or grief. Peter had come to terms with his impending death, and after listening to him, I asked what he wanted to do with the time remaining to him.

"All my life," Peter replied, "people have been doing things for me. Just once, before I die, I'd like to do something for someone else."

It so happened that in two days a group of volunteers would be meeting at the hospice. I invited Peter to come as a guest speaker on the topic of living with cancer. I noticed Mrs. Josslin's slender hands begin to flicker about the neck of her blouse and smooth and stretch the hem of her skirt; she feared that Peter might somehow be hurt by my suggestion. Instead, Peter brightened with enthusiasm. "Of course—and I sure can tell some tales!" he replied.

Early on the scheduled day of the meeting, I phoned Peter to ask him to relax his mind and body. Peter's pain was being controlled by Brompton's Mix, a morphine-based drug which can produce drowsiness. Peter was able to overcome this side effect by 7:00 p.m. When I arrived, he had bounced back. I found Peter to be a man in control of these hours and anxious to get on with his task.

The logistics of moving Peter were difficult, for he no longer had the use of his legs. His brother and I did manage, finally, to lift him from his warm bed to the car. The concerned discussion during the move was stilled when Peter snapped, "Let's go. I'm feeling weak and can only talk for fifteen minutes. You're wasting time discussing something I've decided to do."

After assuring Peter that we would accept whatever time and energy he could give us, we started. At the hospice Peter was greeted by a standing ovation and eighty eyes filled with tears, gratitude and love.

Clearly pleased and suddenly a bit shy, Peter began to speak. An intensity of energy and good will quickly filled the modest little room, and his confidence increased. Peter's voice grew in strength and conviction as he began to describe the feelings of dependency, frustration and inadequacy as a person which so often overwhelmed him.

Much of Peter's talk was unflichingly frank and uncompromising. "Let me tell you what it's like for me to go outside to soak up a little sun. Even when someone *asks* me, do you want to go outside, it's not a simple yes or no. I must consider the other person's inconvenience. Suppose in five minutes I have to go to the bathroom—you know, I can't do that by myself, either. Then someone has to move me back in, and out again. So the real question is not 'Do you want to go outside?' but 'If I go outside, can I stay out there long enough to make it worthwhile for the people taking care of me?' "

For over an hour Peter spoke firmly and rapidly about the stress his illness had caused among family members. The cancer, first diagnosed ten years earlier, had triggered the destruction of his marriage. Peter told of his mother's loving support and help, but also intimated a deep sorrow at compounding the many tribulations his mother had endured. Like many dying people, Peter was determined to say whatever was necessary to help the living understand his experiences and feelings, to give some of his life, which he valued so highly, to the living.

The response to Peter's discussion was electrifying. I have no doubt that his lessons are etched to this day in the memories of all who heard him. Peter was exhausted by the effort, and he slept and rested quietly for several days thereafter. But when I next spoke with him, his first words were, "Oh, Elizabeth, I'm very tired, but thank you for giving me the chance to do the one thing that was really important."

The dying have so much to share with the living. I often hear people say, "I can't think of anything that would be 'right' to say to someone who's dying." The dying need no profound pronouncements, but instead seek honesty and directness. When we serve the needs of the dying, we better understand our own mortality and finite existence. Doing nothing because of our own discomfort with death is a great mistake, for the rewards of doing even a little are great.

Taking a chance—leaping into this work with both feet—will be an enriching experience, I promise you! By helping others through the dying or grief process, we can more firmly put our own priorities in order and truly value every day we live. We can, by observing and participating, sense the master plan of life not only for one person, but for all humanity. Too often the dying feel abandoned; everyone around them fears saying or doing the "wrong" thing. As a result, nothing is said or done and a terrible loneliness sets in. Yet love is our only reason for possessing life, and love means nothing when it is hoarded. The love given by caregivers to the dying is returned tenfold.

Chapter Two

Communication

"Uncle Henry died in June, after a trying ordeal with cancer of the throat. He was cross and ill-tempered especially to Aunt Martha and the rest of the family who had taken care of him for many months. It was a sad and bitter end to his life. I do not understand these kinds of people who seem to turn against their loved ones near the end, making the final days a miserable trial for everyone."

When I received this note from a dear friend, many questions and thoughts came into my mind. In whose eyes was the death "miserable?" Did Uncle Henry, his family, or his friends have any preconceived ideas about how a person with cancer dies? Few know, for instance, that fifty percent of cancer patients experience no pain, and that ten percent have only mild pain. Forty percent, less than half, experience moderate to severe pain.

What issues needed to be resolved between Uncle Henry and his family? Did they have relatives, friends or professionals who supported and helped them through this time? When was the last time these family members said to each other, "I love you, I admire you, I cherish you, I will miss you?" When did Uncle Henry have the opportunity to openly communicate his feelings, anxieties and thoughts about death? And who was listening?

What do we really mean when we say "these kinds of people?" There's an element of separateness here. Uncle Henry's death was anticipated; many illnesses follow a general timetable, ending with death. This family was given the opportunity to prepare. How was the time left with Uncle Henry spent? Perhaps, in trying to protect him from becoming distraught at the approach of his death, the family took away the autonomy which Uncle Henry so desperately needed. His failing body contained a functioning mind which expressed itself in the most effective way it knew. Uncle Henry did the best he could with the time and abilities remaining to him. The grievers surrounding him responded with great anger and bewilderment and were left with agonizing questions, not peacefulness.

While the actual circumstances of this death are unknown to me, Uncle Henry serves as a model of one who, faced with death, realizes he has not come to terms with life. The difficulty inherent in this situation is compounded because the family frequently finds it more difficult to come to terms with the impending death than does the dying person. Family members are almost always the ones who will request the physician to do everything possible to maintain life. They say, "I can't deal with this." What they mean is, "I won't deal with death because it's too painful for me." While the family and medical professionals create a veritable storm of treatment, strategies and decisions designed to extend life, the dying person sits alone in the eye of the hurricane.

While this experience is common, it is not necessary. When the family is involved in the care of the dying person, they more easily come to terms with the death process and their own griefwork. Even if the person cannot be cared for at home, much physical care can be given in the hospital setting by family members. In my experience, the dying person nearly always finds peace with death more easily and more quickly than the family. Spiritual convictions and personal relationships are tested; I have noticed that families and patients initially tend to be angry with God, the medical profession, and the injustice of it all. Eventually, the dying person finds a peaceful state of mind and settles in, but often the family remains in a state of confusion. Those families which succeed in expressing their love for each other and the dying person are families which are able to accept the transition of death, let go of what was, and go forward with life as an everchanging experience.

Strong emotions are usually exhibited when the person is first told of a life-threatening illness. Individuals grapple with these feelings, develop their own coping mechanisms, and then become comfortable with them. All goes well until the physician tells them the disease has progressed despite intensive treatment, or that it has reappeared. Once more strong emotions come forth, often including questions like, "Why? I did everything the doctor told me!"

By the time the patient realizes that the disease has progressed beyond medical knowledge, generally he has come to accept that whatever time is left should be used to prepare for death. I have been told by colleagues that someone who has no religious beliefs struggles more with the concept of death than does the person who has a strong concept of God. This may be true, but among those I have observed who believe death is simply a total cessation of body and soul, the peacefulness exhibited at the end mirrored that of the believers.

Elisabeth Kubler-Ross, M.D., has written guidelines to help us better understand this process called death. Her five stages, widely publicized, have been used and abused to the point where caregivers often categorize the dying person, trapping him or her in a series of boxes marked "denial, anger, bargaining, depression or acceptance," expecting the patient to follow along in a tidy emotional sequence. This boxing up of the person who has not yet died is premature; the feelings, desires, and spirit of the individual are in full force so long as life remains. The categories identified by Kübler-Ross have been constructed to make death seem an intellectual process; in fact, advanced academic degrees in death and dying are now being offered at some colleges and universities. The truth is that dying is the least scientific work any of us will ever do.

Patients and families experience the five stages of death in different order, jump backward and forward from one to another, and stay in each one for as long as is necessary. As a caregiver, one must not interfere with this process. The pressure on a patient or family to achieve acceptance is often the result of the caregiver's need, not theirs.

As a counselor, I often see family communication break down as a direct result of the stress of a life-threatening illness. As a general rule, if the lines of communication were open during good health, they will remain open throughout the more intense relationship during illness. Unfortunately, the opposite is also true. A lack of communication before illness usually invites limited communication after a diagnosis such as cancer. During my two years as a chemotherapist, I was with patients from time of diagnosis through remission, cure or death. I was able to work with seriously ill people and their families to emphasize the importance of sharing feelings in a non-threatening way. When the going got tough for these people, many managed to talk about most of their problems and feelings. While years of family interaction cannot be changed in a few weeks or months—or even should be changed—the patience and love of a caregiver can often help a family improve or avoid an intolerable situation.

Who sets the tone for this scenario called dying? The players usually include the medical team, family, friends and perhaps a spiritual leader. The central figure is the dying person. Who has control at this time? The physician, the keeper of knowledge? The family, who doesn't want to be separated from the loved one? The clergyman, who feels a responsibility to give leadership and spiritual comfort? All the friends who had friends who went through the same thing?

I have seen each of the above take the leading role. But whose death is this? What happens when the patient takes charge and decides, perhaps, "No more chemotherapy," or "I want Cousin Terry to take care of my affairs, not Uncle Alex"? Do the family, friends, and clergy come unglued? The dying person should be setting the tone for this entire drama, and too often is not allowed to do so. When the dying person selects the tone, theme, and leading players in this last scene, a sense of closure is more likely to be achieved. And the dying person may choose someone to take that central role, or may keep it.

A flood of vital concerns and questions arise during illness, and the patient is quite likely to acquire unfortunate misunderstandings regarding the nature of the disease. A caregiver who is mindful of the whole person can do much to dispel these clouds of doubt.

I worked with a man who was convalescing from successful surgery to arrest cancer of the colon. Derek was a bachelor in his early fifties, a professor at a large Southern university who was widely respected for his research and scholarship. Derek bore the diagnosis and surgery with as much courage as he could muster, and continued to take the prescribed medications after his return home.

While at his home, Derek developed painful and puzzling symptoms; uncontrolled tearing of his eyes, a limp numbness in his arm, and a very rough and dry skin. Frightened that the cancer had reccurred, Derek was given a battery of tests. The results indicated *no* cancer present.

But, because of his physician's travel plans, Derek was not informed immediately. His fears multiplying, Derek leaped to the conclusion that the news must be the worst. One day he found in his mailbox an envelope from his physician. In it was the entire text of the test report. As a college professor, Derek certainly had the knowledge to decipher the test results or contact someone who could. Years of education and experience, however, do not insulate us from our fear of illness. It was not a calm, cool professor who tore that envelope open; it was a frightened man who felt alone and threatened by something inside him which he could not control.

Derek's eyes flew rapidly over the text of the report, picking up a word here or there, until he reached the final sentence in the last paragraph: "The symptoms exhibited are the result of chemotherapy versus disease progression." In reality, the conclusion of the report meant that the symptoms were the result of chemotherapy—not of disease reoccurrence. No disease was found. Chemotherapy was causing Derek's symptoms.

Derek, however, felt as though his every fear was confirmed. He interpreted the report to mean that his symptoms were caused by chemotherapy struggling against the progression of the disease. His doctor had been so impressed with Derek's intellectual control that he had not reckoned with the tremendous power of Derek's emotions. When faced with a statement his intellect could not immediately decipher, Derek's feelings of fear and devastation boiled over.

He called me, weeping and repeating over and over again, "I told you something was wrong. I just knew it." It took a good deal of emotional reassurance and repetition of facts to convince him of the truth of the report.

After the crisis was over, Derek mentioned how important it had been for him to be able to share his fears with a person whose voice and caring he recognized and who had the time to explain until he understood. By the way, he has remained free of the disease that caused a life crisis and re-evaluation.

Caregivers can also encourage more open communication and mutual respect among the dying and medical personnel. Meetings between small groups of nurses and four or five patients are often useful. At one particularly memorable meeting, a certain young woman, Pat, opened the discussion by asking, "Why don't nurses seem to really care about us? I mean *really* care?" Pat was a bright and well-educated woman in her thirties whose degenerating heart was that of an eighty-year-old. She had worked through most of her feelings about having a life which would be shorter and more restricted than those of her friends. However, depression and anxiety often preoccupied her. While these subjects were not in the least unusual in the meetings, I was startled by the vehemence of her question.

"What is it that makes you think nurses don't care,

Pat?" I asked. The nurses in the room shifted uneasily, looking a bit confused and hurt.

"Because they never act like it," Pat snapped. "On a normal day, one comes in the room with my medications. 'How are you today?' I'm asked, and then she doesn't wait to hear what I have to say in response to her routine question. I may feel lousy, but she surely doesn't want to hear about it. I take the pills, and she's out the door. Another comes in to take my blood pressure and temperature. Then another, and another. And of this whole parade, not one says more than the first one did. Sometimes, if one does stop to talk, and I tell her something in confidence, like what I'm thinking about, she'll write it in the chart. Then everybody knows. My doctor asks me about it. I feel betrayed."

Silence filled the room. Then Rita, one of the younger nurses, spoke out, "Oh, Pat, didn't anyone tell you we use team nursing here?" Pat shook her head. "Well," she continued, "team nursing means that one nurse gives the medications to everyone on the floor. That's her job, her assignment for the day, and it is totally her responsibility. Another takes the morning readings. Each nurse has a different assignment every morning. I'll bet you are used to having one nurse take care of all your needs. The same familiar face to answer your call light. That's called primary nursing."

Before Pat could respond, another nurse added: "Yes. And if we see or hear something that we think might affect your recovery, we're obligated to note it on your chart. If you're depressed, I'll write that.

Some of the drugs you're taking can cause depression, and my notes might be a signal to your doctor that your medication should be re-evaluated."

"Okay, but why do you have to bustle around so coldly? What about my feelings?" asked Pat.

As the conversation continued and other patients chimed in with similar emotions, the nurses realized that patients truly needed not only explanations of what to expect in the hospital, but also some individual attention and genuine empathy. Both groups realized that the nurses' staffing structure—which nurses could not control—worked against patients who felt lonely and needed someone to share their feelings.

As a result of the meeting—and others which followed—nursing in that hospital took on a warmer tone. Even during times of staff shortages, nurses agreed that disciplining themselves to respect the emotional needs of patients yielded a deeper satisfaction in their work. Many had missed a more traditional primary nursing strategy, but felt powerless to overcome the structure of team nursing.

Pat's challenge resulted in understanding and growth not only for the patients, but for nurses, too. Many benefitted from her boldness. Pat spoke well for the dying person, who often feels that the progress of the disease destroys not only the physical self, but their humanity as well.

Nurses Caroline M. Arnold and Patricia M. Ismert became deeply attuned to the feelings and experiences of people dying in hospitals. The following are their words.

REFLECTIONS OF A PATIENT

Inside my body is a person—Me! Please listen to me, feel with me and for me. Although I am sometimes helpless, treat me as an adult. Don't make me submit like a child to bewildering routines. Please preserve my now-fragile dignity, enable me to keep my self-respect. Don't strip me of my identity when you strip me of my clothes. Don't make me beg for relief of pain. Don't act as if I'm stupid because I don't know about my body or treat my body like a machine in a repair shop. I beg you to remember that illness, pain, and fear bring on overly emotional and sometimes seemingly unreasonable behavior. These unknown surroundings bewilder me. When you remain a stranger to me, my fears may cause me to behave in a manner even more unreasonable. Look at me when you speak to me. Listen to what I'm saying. Come and speak to me, even briefly, just so I know I am not forgotten. I cannot stand total lack of concern. Give me tender loving care.

Make the things you must do to me more bearable. Call me by name, tell me who you are, touch me. Tell me what you are going to do—even though you've told me before. The sound of your voice, the feel of your touch reminds me that I am not alone. Show me your compassion, let me see it in your face, and hear it in your voice. Let me know by your gentle, caring touch. Show me that you care enough to know about me. Show me, through your care, that I am a person.

Don't take away my privacy when you intrude in your helpful way to care for me. Everything is so open here—and I am a very private person. Knock on my door before you enter my room. Pull the curtains a-round my bed. Cover me when you bathe me. Keep my door closed if I request it.

You see, I bring not only my sick body to you, I bring my total being. I am a suffering human being. Think not only of my body but also of my spirit. Offer me spiritual care. Pray with me or for me. Cry with me if you feel the need, for you may be my closest friend at that moment. You can make my life bearable until my family or someone important to me arrives. I am weak, fragile, and vulnerable. Help me to be strong.

Respect me, even though my body is wrinkled with age or made unsightly by disease. Don't abandon me and leave me like a helpless prisoner. Don't isolate me with your rituals. When I feel your discomfort, it's easy to feel lonely in the hospital. My day becomes bleak and gray.

Outside my door many disembodied voices call to each other. Your laughter and joy make me long to be included. Oh, how I need someone to laugh with, to share joy with. The constant paging...who are those people? Carts clatter by my door. I hear never-ending klinking, clatter, bumps, and rattles that no one ex-plains. I am bombarded with noise when one of my greatest needs is to be quiet.

Give me tender loving care so that I will not be so fearful. Then I know that you will help make the suf-fering bearable and keep hope alive so that some joy may enter my life again. Knowing this will make my days brighter and my nights shorter.

Chapter Three

Serve Simply

To "serve simply" means honoring decisions made by the patient which, had the caregiver been given the choice, might have been very different ones. The ability to participate in the care of a seriously ill person without judging the behavior or actions of that person or others surrounding the situation is a skill which requires constant conscious practice to refine.

To develop a nonjudgemental attitude, remember that while the ill person is the focus of the caregiver's attention, he or she may not be that person the caregiver most values. Love, faith, and human kindness are the ideals to which the caregivers aspires, regardless of the varieties of emotions, illnesses, or situations which may be rendered day by day. Letting go of assumptions, prejudices, judgements, and conditional love is an important priority for caregivers. The ill person and his or her family is the focus of the benefits of the caregiver's personal growth in this regard. Work with the dying is also work on yourself! What you bring into a situation is not what you know, but who you are.

The focus of the caregiver should be on the physical

and emotional well-being of the patient. There is continuing debate concerning specific medication for the terminally ill. As a caregiver, I am in favor of the quality of life as opposed to engaging in treatments which are sometimes painful, disturbing, costly, and futile in all ways, not just in preventing death.

This sort of debate is becoming more public as medical science advances into new realms of research. While others debate, however, the caregiver can *do*, making manifest values and beliefs which are abstract to others.

Taking action, however, is not always without a conflict. I have learned that it is more important to do what is right than to do what is easiest. When a man named Ted called and asked me to help him prepare for death spiritually and emotionally, I felt it right that I should.

Ted had spent six painful months in and out of the hospital. The quality time he had bargained for had come and gone; cancer had invaded his internal organs, and there was no hope for his recovery. Our hope was concentrated on a peaceful death which he would control.

After forty-eight years of hard living, Ted began to make peace with God and anticipate his death. His room was prepared; relaxing music was played, the draperies were kept open to allow the sun to enter. Ted's cat had a special place next to him and friends and relatives came and went. When I shared with Ted my beliefs about the death process and the afterlife, he looked rather surprised.

"Those are all the things I have been dreaming about, and sometimes I see friends who have already died," he responded.

As part of our preparation for Ted's death, I asked his wife to repeat frequently: "You are surrounded by the pure white light. Nothing but good shall come to you and nothing but good shall go from you," both for her own comfort and for Ted's. She was to verbally encourage him toward the light he would perceive while dying, reminding him not to look to the left nor to the right, but to go directly to the light.

On the following Monday, while he was alone, Ted pulled the intravenous tube from his arm. An imbalance of sodium followed quickly, and Ted became totally irrational, even when the I.V. was restarted. Ted was comatose most of the time from that point on.

Even though Ted was no longer responsive, every day that I saw him I shared more of my interpretations and feelings about death. Death would be a peaceful experience, I emphasized, and he would be aware of it all. Ted requested that his body not be touched for several hours after death so all the life forces could leave it and enter the astral body which becomes active at the time of death. He shared with me the belief that the astral body, or soul, goes through several phases after death. This is the time we evaluate our growth on the physical, or earthly plane, judging ourselves. It's a time for awakening spiritually. There is no physical pain involved.Finally, just before the silver cord is severed and clinical death is complete, the soul experiences the sensation of floating, of lightness, of letting go. I continued to soothe Ted's apparent physical discomforts as much as possible, while assuring him that he had no reason to fear death.

Just before Ted died, the family's cat slipped out the back door. She was a well-loved cat, unaccustomed to being outside, and Ted's wife and children hurried outside to catch her. While the family searched, Ted gained consciousness and sat up on the side of the bed.

"I'm ready," he said softly to his wife when she returned, out of breath. These were his last words. Ted died early the next morning, his wife holding him in her arms.

I felt at peace with Ted's passing. He chose to set himself on the path to the next life, which meant turning away from the path of this life. To Ted, choosing meant a great deal. For those of us surrounding Ted, his choice was, as always, respected.

Some two weeks or so after Ted's death, I had a dream which I believe was a significant message to me from Ted. In the dream, my home was a luxuriant garden filled with sensuous colors and aromas. Friends and relatives had gathered; the women wore dresses in the clean, bright colors of flowers, and their wide-brimmed hats cast deep shadows over their faces and throats. I did not know exactly who the people were, but their voices and vibrations formed a soothing murmur which cast peacefulness throughout my garden home.

In my dream I also had a husband, but his face was turned away from me. I touched his hand and said, "It is time for me to die. Let us go inside."

I still could not see his face as he led me to my lovely bedroom with windows to the garden and a canopied bed. I lay down and he covered me with a cloud-soft quilt. I thought of my death, without fear, and thought of my husband and all our time together, without any regret of having to let go.

I looked deeply into my husband's eyes, giving his hand one last squeeze. The man next to me was Ted.

I believe the message for me in the dream was of caring, support, and encouragement. It was verification that after his death, all was well with Ted's soul. Death can be just as you choose it to be: a beautiful experience, being consciously aware of every moment, or a struggle with letting go of who you think you are, using drugs to make the pain go away, and missing the final curtain because of fear.

Finally, serving simply means to allow the ill person to set the pace and level of the care needed. It is important that the caregiver's needs and expectations stay out of the way. We who are not now facing our own death sometimes have difficulty distinguishing among varieties of hope; we must recognize that hoping the dying person gets well again is simply wasted energy. On the other hand, hope for an easy and peaceful death is a strong and encouraging hope for the dying. Praying for healing of the body and spirit, knowing that death does not indicate whether the prayers were unanswered, can be a very powerful and positive channeling of a caregiver's energy.

While the caregiver may grieve over the changed visage of the ill person—and this grief is real—it is the need of the dying person which should determine if a wig or make-up should be worn; who shall visit and how often, and dozens of other things. It is appropriate to hope that these decisions are respected by all, and that they are implemented. Above all, it is also appropriate to hope for one's own strength and understanding, and for the ability to stay consistent with one's values and ideals.

To serve simply is the caregiver's goal. Through consistent dedication, the caregiver will participate in one of life's most mysterious and intimate experiences.

Chapter Four

Learning To Care

The needs of the dying are many. Sustained and expert medical attention is necessary, if only to relieve the symptoms of the illness. The services of clergy, lawyers, and other professionals may be required. The dying need assurances of being loved and cared for; they appreciate the presence of family, friends, neighbors and associates.

But, thus surrounded by well-meaning people ready to decide every question, medical and otherwise, the terminally-ill can easily lose those rights and abilities that others take for granted; the right to privacy and quiet, to move about, to spend time with one's chosen companions, and to be fully informed about one's illness. Weakened and vulnerable, they may not be able to summon the strength to demand access to a telephone to call a friend or to walk from one room to another.

A caregiver who lovingly and respectfully focuses attention on the most simple of human rights and needs serves both the body and the soul of the patient. Too often, friends, relatives, and medical personnel concentrate on the disease, not on the person.

The condition of the ailing heart or liver or lungs can become the chief topic of daily conversation swirling around the dying person. A caregiver who can draw closer and focus on the wants and needs expressed by the patient may learn that his or her top priority is finding out who won last night's bowling tournament or getting someone to change the station on the radio. Listening with the heart yields many ways to help the dying.

In my experience, the dying fear most three things: pain, abandonment, and helplessness. Together, these factors form a demanding challenge to the caregiver. They cannot always be overcome, but a compassionate caregiver can give much-appreciated, if not entire, relief from these difficulties inherent in serious illness and death.

One of the first things that can be done is to try to stop the pain of the patient. The medical team will most likely control the physical pain, although some doctors remain haunted by fear of the patient becoming addicted, and so refuse to prescribe narcotics for effective pain control until "the end" is near. Caregivers need to learn to be nonjudgemental about the pain the individual may experience; that is, to control their responses and concentrate on loving and caring for the person without letting the pain interfere with the quality of that care.

When a caregiver becomes overly-concerned with the physical pain of the patient, the pain will become accentuated in that person's mind. In either focusing upon the pain or attempting to deny its strength, the caregiver communicates this concern by voice and facial expressions. Then the patient must bear a double burden: the pain, and the caregiver's feelings about it.

It is far better for a caregiver to focus on love, peacefulness, and the human needs of the ill person. By concentrating on these positive qualities, the caregiver can relieve the burden of pain on the patient rather than adding to it.

The pain of seriously ill people often worsens during holiday periods, particularly in December. During these times, chemotherapy seems to cause more side effects, symptoms become more annoying, and medications appear to be less effective.

I believe these phenomena are emotional pain manifested as physical pain. They stem from the dying person's wish that everything would once again be as before the illness, and from the disappointment which results from realizing how impossible this wish is. I have felt the disappointment as a survivor. Since my father's death, Christmas has not been my favorite time of the year. I, too, longed for what could not be, instead of exploring the existing potential of the day. I especially wanted Christmas to be the same as when Dad was living. Instead, year after year, the holiday got worse; each Christmas I used alcohol to numb my pain. It didn't work, of course. I eventually had to confront the source of my pain and overcome it in a positive way. So must the dying confront the reality of disease and deal with both the physical and the emotional pain, recognizing the source of that pain and devising a way to overcome it.

This is not to say that a caregiver should be insensitive to physical pain. It is a part of many illnesses and may serve as an indicator of complications or other physical changes. Pain where none is expected can signal other problems as well. As a hospice worker, I once spent a good deal of time trying to figure out why not one of several medications, all very powerful, had helped a cancer patient's pain. Finally, the man's wife confessed to withholding the drugs. She had been torn by religious beliefs that forbade medications; she could not bring herself to give them to her husband, though his beliefs were different. We solved the problem by providing a hospice volunteer to dispense the drugs daily, thus relieving the husband's pain and the wife's guilt.

Those who are seriously ill or dying often realize that the pain they feel is not entirely physical. A nurse who was suffering from acute high blood pressure, acquired perhaps from the stresses of her job, once commented bitterly to me: "My doctor is giving me a new tranquilizer to teach me how to cope with this." In other words, the real source of her pain, the enormous stresses of her speciality as practiced in that hospital, had not been alleviated. Her feelings about her work situation and her illness were not being explored. Instead of being helped down the more difficult but more fruitful path of confronting and resolving the conflicts she felt, the nurse's feelings were being deadened and shoved aside. As much as this woman needed medication to control her high blood pressure, she needed help to deal with a situation which aggravated the illness. Besides top-notch medical care, she needed equally good care from a caregiver who could listen, advise, and gather information from her.

Simple techniques can be used to help ease the pain and anxiety of seriously ill or dying patients. While working as a chemotherapy nurse, I learned how important a pleasant environment can be. Chemotherapy is often a painful process; it hurts no less to be stuck with a needle the ninetieth time than it does the first. People who are already ill don't look forward to the side effects, such as nausea and itching, which so often result. Consequently, "Elizabeth's room," where chemotherapy was given, was not the most popular place in the clinic, but I was able to improve even this room's ambience and, thus, the patient's experience in it.

First, the room was painted a lively yellow, a high energy color. Instead of the usual lab-type chairs, I had two comfortable recliners brought in, as well as green plants and colorful posters. One of my favorite posters was a photo of a road disappearing into a truly breathtaking Southwestern sunset. The caption read: "Life is not a destination, but a journey." A stereo with headphones and a small collection of records with stress-reducing music completed the renovation.

This homelike, cheerful atmosphere allowed many patients to be treated without undue stress. A patient could come in, relax and put his feet up, chat a bit, select a recording, put on the headphones, and drift easily with the music. Although the unpleasant side effects of the drugs still occurred, they seemed less intense and easier to bear.

A great challenge to the chemotherapy nurse is to find a suitable vein in people who have weak or "burned" veins as a result of extended therapy. When treating such a person, I would sit in the other recliner and play the music aloud. Then both of us would relax, close our eyes, and imagine the veins growing as big as tree trunks. Frequently, I could then give the medication without difficulty.

The chemotherapy room was peaceful and filled with encouragement. Although people didn't like their reasons for being there, most eventually became quite comfortable with it.

The positive influence of an attractive environment for a dying person extends to home care, too, where it is often easier to accomplish. I suggest placing the bed in the middle of the living room or family room, where most of the family activities go on. A hospital bed is the right height for easy care of the sick person and for linen changes, but some prefer their own beds, set up on blocks, rather than an unfamiliar electrical contraption. Siderails are a sensible safety factor, but should be lowered whenever possible during the day; lying behind siderails often makes one feel helpless and isolated. While drawsheets should always be used to make linen changes easier, the sheets and blankets should be colorful. Personal items can be placed near the bed—photos of loved ones, favorite books, this or that momento of a special time of life. In setting up the patient's bed, remember that the sun gives energy; place the bed so that the occupant can bathe in it.

The ill person may prefer the privacy of the bedroom at various times during or throughout the illness. If so, a call system must be devised. A buzzer, bell, or whistle is effective so long as strength remains to use it. Beyond this, all the other principles apply: sunshine, color, and company are needed, as are other affirmations of the importance of the patient. Music and meditation exercises are inspiring and can be useful in easing pain and anxiety. A spiritual picture or beautiful landscape can be an effective point of concentration when placed at eye level on an opposite wall.

Fluffy down-filled pillows tucked all around the body and used to support aching joints and limbs also soothe the patient. The warmth generated by draping warm wet towels over the body and then adding plastic sheeting and blankets can relieve both mental and physical pain and anxiety.

Fear of abandonment also besets the seriously ill person. From the time the illness is diagnosed, the patient is aware of the changes in attitude of friends, family and others. In addition, the person may find in ternal shifts in priorities which are as dramatic as the changes in appearance, strength, and abilities which accompany illness. It is the exceptionally secure and self-confident individual who, under these circumstances, does not ask, silently or aloud, "Who will stay

with me through this ordeal? Which of my relationships will collapse under the strain of all these
changes? Which will hold up?"

The dying may feel these fears confirmed when certain friends or relatives become "too busy" to spend
time at the bedside. Sorrow, loneliness, and bewilderment spring forth as the dying person questions his or
her own worth—"Have I become intolerably revolting
because of this sickness?" The entire worth of the relationship may be examined: "Did she ever really love
me? Was it faked all those years?"

Those who studiously avoid the dying may do so
out of ignorance and fear of their own mortality, which
they see reflected in the face of the dying person. Having once been overpowered by such feelings, I know
them well. Some people cannot be persuaded to respond to the dying person's request for company, but
many can. Regardless of the caregiver's success in
contacting these recalcitrants, it helps to explain to
the ill person that the problem lies in the fear of the
avoider, not in any aspect of the patient or the illness.
We tend to push away self-confrontations, and feel
more comfortable by avoiding them completely.

To ease the fear of abandonment, the caregiver
may first arrange to keep comforting personal mo-
mentos near the patient as reminders of the importance of the life which is still being lived. Reinforce
the affirmation of life by introducing children and
pets, blooming plants, perhaps colorful tropical fish.
All these have the capacity to cheer the dying along
with companionship and an important sense of to-

getherness with living things.

There are many ways of preventing the ill person from being overwhelmed by the fear of abandonment. After I had been badly injured in a nearly-fatal automobile accident, I learned firsthand how comforting it was to have friends bring in dinner and make it a real event with candlelight, soft music, and my favorite incense. My daughter came to visit me for two weeks. What a luxury her company was! Friends helped me attend meetings, go for a drive, and kept me informed of the local goings-on. The memory of such special care and concern remains precious to me. While it would have been easy for my friends to lose contact over my long recovery period, many put forth special effort to keep me from feeling abandoned.

While contact with the ill or dying person ought to be regular, it need not be elaborate. During times when the patient is exhausted, depressed, or hurting, a simple holding of the hand or gentle stroking of the brow is very effective, and perhaps as much as the person wants.

The caregiver must listen with the heart to learn how much contact is wanted. Sometimes, a large gathering of family and friends may cause overwhelming expectations in the dying person. In other cases, such a gathering brings only pleasure. The habits and personality traits of the patient prior to the illness will be a clue to the caregiver, for they generally remain constant throughout the illness.

Some dying people enjoy company and the reassurance of loved ones right up until death. One such person was Catherine, a dear woman who was in chemotherapy for a year before it was discovered the cancer had permeated many of her organs. After considering all possible options, Catherine chose to put her affairs in order, spend the remainder of her life as comfortably as she could, and prepare for her death. The morning of the day she died, I asked what more I could do to make her comfortable.

"You'd better call my lawyer," she said. "I revised my will and I need to sign it. He's supposed to bring it this afternoon, but I don't think there's time to wait."

After I took care of that, Catherine motioned me over to the bed. I held her hand and cradled her arm. "One more thing—I have a dear friend, Susie; we've been friends since childhood. I'd really like to see her today. Do you think the way I look now would upset her?"

I responded that I thought her friend would be happy to see her again and share in the death, good looks or not.

"Our parents were good friends," Catherine continued, "and while they visited, Susie and I got into the homemade blackberry brandy." She chuckled at her memories. "We did have some fun!"

Pleasant recollections of Susie, family and other friends poured forth as Catherine related other pleasurable experiences of her lifetime. When the lawyer arrived with the will, I slipped out of the room to phone Susie. With Catherine's doctor's encouragement, I asked Susie if she might happen to have any blackberry brandy to share with Catherine one more time. She responded with obvious delight. "I'm out of blackberry, but I've just finished making some raspberry brandy. Will that do?"

"Close enough!" I replied, and Susie was on her way over. That afternoon, a surprised and delighted Catherine sipped raspberry brandy, sharing old times once again with her good friend. She was at peace with herself and her impending death. During the night, after her sister-in-law arrived to say good-bye, Catherine died peacefully and quietly.

To try to deal with a person's fear of abandonment by becoming overly-solicitous may be counter-productive. Some people require more privacy and quiet time as death approaches. The caregiver must be sensitive to this often unspoken need. I am reminded of the father of a large and closely-knit family who kept vigil by his bed day and night. The atmosphere was intense as family members prayed, wept, spoke what they believed to be their last words ever to their dad, and—I sensed—kept him from gliding easily into the next plane of consciousness.

As a hospice caregiver, I was at length able to persuade the family to take a respite from their intense involvement with their father's death. "You need a rest, he needs a rest," I urged.

As the family agreed that having dinner at a nice restaurant might be a good thing to do, one person asked, "What if Dad dies while we're gone?"

"What if? What will you do? How will you feel if that happens?" I responded gently.

The ensuing discussion led to a consensus that perhaps Dad, who had been somewhat of a private person all his life, would appreciate the privacy, and that if he did die, family members would feel some regret, but no catastrophic sense of having failed. I reiterated my firm belief that many choose the exact time of their death, and that their father ought to be given the option of slipping away without fanfare.

As it happened, the father did choose to die after family members had returned to his room, kissed him, assured him of their return, and left for the restaurant. The family, having been prepared, handled the passing well. They asked me many times to describe exactly how his death took place, saying, "Did he have any last words?" Soon, however, they were able to get on with their lives without feeling guilt about "abandoning" their dad when he needed them most. Actually, what he needed most was the space in which to take the next step in the life/death cycle.

The clergy is another source of support for the dying. Many seriously ill people find great comfort in discussions with the clergy and look forward to such visits. Some who have had unhappy experiences with bombastic, condemning interpretations of religion may be receptive to other interpretations which focus instead on a message of God's non-judgemental love. They may thus enjoy talking to a clergyman who shares that emphasis. But if the dying person totally and consistently rejects any suggestion of contact with the clergy—or anyone else for that matter—then the caregiver must respect this wish.

When assuring the dying person of dependable and

constant support, it is important that the caregiver bear in mind that the dying person's wishes be carefully heard, for the caregiver can, in a determination to do the most possible good, inadvertently let his or her own idea of what is good for the dying person dominate the strategy.

Such conflicting notions often surface over the issue of food. From infancy we equate giving food with caring. In addition, we believe food always gives strength: "Here, eat something, you'll feel better," we urge on ill person. The dying, however, reach a point when food is not wanted, and no amount of cajoling or tempting will change that fact.

The caregiver may not want to hear the message that food and water are no longer needed. It conflicts with the idea that the person is being supported and cared for, not left to die. One caregiver, a wife caring for her husband, became obsessed with making sure her husband ate three meals a day, whether or not the food was wanted. Although the husband was in a nursing home where nourishing meals were provided, the wife cooked her husband's every meal at home and carried it in. Then she fed her husband. If he refused to eat, the wife begged and badgered him to eat bite after bite. It was a genuine—and genuinely painful—battle of wills, and the caregiver's good intentions only heightened the intensity of it.

One day the wife brought a slice of lovely chocolate cake for her husband's dessert. "See this cake I brought you, dear. Isn't it your favorite?" she began, advancing the loaded fork to her husband's face.

"I don't want it," the old man said.

"Just a bite, it's so good, I made it just for you."

"I don't want it."

As the chocolate cake came ever closer and the wife's hand touched her husband's jaw to urge him to open his mouth, the old man's heart stopped. To his wife's horror, the husband simply chose to die, right then and there, rather than eat that piece of chocolate cake.

In contrast, Gramp's family, the Jurys, dealt with his refusal to eat quite differently. One day Gramp removed his dentures and announced that he would eat or drink no more. After he had become comatose, the family decided that if Gramp preferred to refuse all food and liquids, they were not going to defy his wishes by forcing him to eat.

To the caregiver, seeing a dying person make this decision and carry it out may be a wrenching experience because of vivid images of what "starving to death" means. Yet in all my experience with the dying, I have found that "starving" is an issue only if the caregiver makes it so. For the dying, it's a comfortable and seemingly natural way of letting go of the earthly body. Through this difficult aspect of the illness, the caregiver must remain loyal to the real needs of the patient.

Helplessness during illnesses is dreaded by all seriously ill people, but for many it is a necessary evil which must be finally accepted. It is not easy for a person to find it necessary to ask for a drink of water, to be helped to the bathroom, to have a pillow moved or blanket turned back for comfort—and it's even more difficult to have to wait when these needs are immediate. Anger born of frustration with one's own weakness can explode toward those very people who are trying to be helpful the most.

Caregivers can prevent the ill person from panicking about helplessness by making the most frequently-needed objects and equipment accessible to the person who is able to reach and grasp objects. Water ought to be within reach at all times, and a portable commode may be very useful. Care must be taken to regularly check the placement of equipment and supplies. I remember one particularly infuriating morning while I was recovering from the car accident. I was about to take my crutches, get out of bed, and use a portable commode placed near, but not near enough, my bed. As I eased myself onto the commode, my crutches slipped and fell out of reach. I was not close enough to use the bed to support myself, and holler as I might, I could not awaken my daughter, Debi, in the room down the hall.

The vision of my impotent fury there on the little commode is laughable now, because my helplessness was temporary. For the terminally ill, however, this is a serious problem. My situation really required a buzzer, bell, or even a walkie-talkie system to alert Debi to my distress. A long hooked pole or cane would have helped me reach my crutches.

Thoughtfulness and a bit of ingenuity can go a long way to help a seriously ill person maintain independence and dignity.

The telephone is critical to communication for ill people. Put the bed by the phone or the phone by the bed. Frequently-called numbers, written larger, should be taped on the phone. I've also found it gratifying to be able to turn *off* the phone's ringing one way or another, so that a private conversation or much-needed nap is not interrupted. As wireless phones become less and less expensive, they are also becoming smaller and lighter—a real boon to those who are weak or cannot hear a regular phone.

There are, of course, some things the ill person cannot do. When I was hospitalized, many friends helped me maintain feelings of independence by doing many things for me. Mother helped me bathe, knowing that feeling clean had been important to me all my life. Donna gave me a lovely pedicure and some white Sangria. Susan washed my hair, Ed and Mike gave me healing energy, and one of the women I'd helped care for as a nurse brought homemade cookies. One gift was a beautiful mobile of butterflies which was hung over my bed. It was so finely balanced that even a puff of my breath while I lay flat on my back sent it gently floating about, giving me quiet, restful pleasure.

All of these gifts of both time and substance were given in the spirit of loving willingness. I felt not helpless, but simply humanly helped when Donna trimmed and filed my toenails, chatting along with the latest news. The cookies were excellent because they'd been baked to share. And the mobile was a source of entertainment and fantasy which I myself could control without noise or distraction.

The combination of my caregivers' helpful and supportive attitudes and the efficiency of their care made me feel *helped*, not helpless.

To "serve simply" means to focus on those things which matter most to the ill person. Few who are dying expect or desire profound statements or heroic efforts on their behalf. What matters most is the here and now, and the venting of emotions. Most of us have been so conditioned that we must verbalize our thoughts and feelings if we are to be understood; in truth, the non-verbal aspects of communication are the most intimate and sincere. Loving and respecting a person through the ups and downs of illness plants a seed of love, a seed which will grow and yield even more love.

When I am with a dying person, I often simply say, "What can I do for you today to make it just a little bit better?" The request which follows may be to draw the blinds or open the draperies, help the person from bed to chair, fetch writing paper, or bring the phone within reach. Sometimes the requests are more complicated, but they are nearly always asked for in the same spirit of simplicity and comfort.

It is this simple doing—this caring process—for which caregivers take responsibility. We cannot be responsible for the ultimate results, which are influenced by, and perhaps dependent upon, factors we cannot know or control. The caregiver's work goes on in an atmosphere of the highly-charged emotions of at least one and probably several others. And there are circumstances which sometimes cannot be known or felt beforehand. The illness itself is not predictable. But the caregiver must go forward with faith, respect, and love, putting in motion a process which is intended to make the ill person's day "just a little bit better."

The importance of the loving process over unpredictable results was made clear to me when I worked with Tom, a man dying of chronic obstructive pulmonary disease. He was hospitalized, and his life was measured in days.

While spending a little time with Tom one day, I noticed a small stuffed possum on his bedside table. I asked about it and what it meant to him.

"Look at the pictures under that book,"he said.

While reaching for the pictures, I also noticed that his reading material was entitled, *A Dieter's Guide to Weight Loss During Sex*.

When I chuckled at the title, Tom said, "I couldn't think of a better way to go than laughing over one of those jokes," and began to recite his favorites. Looking at the pictures underneath the book, I realized that the little stuffed animal represented Tom's pet possum, Opie.

One photograph showed a lanky, sunbrowned Tom and beady-eyed Opie together on a campout. In another, newly-bathed Opie was posing sleek and shiny, his bushy fur properly fluffed up. Clearly, Opie and Tom had a delightful and very close relationship. As I glanced at Tom's face, I saw a longing for that little beast, for the good times they'd had together.

Knowing it is often more successful to ask for one's

supervisor's forgiveness later than for permission beforehand, I suggested to Tom that we might be able to
bring Opie into the hospital for one last visit.

"Really?" grinned Tom, his eyes open wide. "How?"

I had acquired quite a bit of experience in getting
cats and small dogs up to hospital rooms, so I suggested that one of Tom's friends bring the little possum in a basket. I was somewhat concerned that the
animal remain securely in Tom's room and not slip
out the door. I knew how startling a Pekinese dog run-
ning down the hall could be to the good people who
worked at the hospital, let alone how they might feel
about a possum! Nonetheless, we arranged with
Tom's friend to bring Opie to the hospital for one last
visit later that night. Tom, while weak and emaciated,
was radiant with happiness and anticipation. Satisfied that I had helped make this day better for him, I
went on with my routine.

It wasn't until several weeks later that I learned the
outcome of our plan. A nurse who had cared for Tom
told me the rest of the story. Tom's friend had indeed
put Opie into the basket for the hospital visit. On the
way, however, Opie escaped from the basket and was
run over by a car. Tom, waiting to see his beloved pet,
was bitterly disappointed and overwhelmed with
grief when he learned of Opie's death. Tom died the
next morning without happiness, and very much alone.

Upon hearing this, my heart sank like a stone. On
reflection, however, I chose to learn a difficult lesson
from Tom and Opie. I could not control the circumstances. I did not imagine that Opie could so easily

escape the basket.

To continue my work, I had to choose to not agonize over what had happened. The plan was conceived in hope and love, but the results were influenced by factors which I could not anticipate. Rather than accept a paralysis born of the fear of making a mistake, I chose to continue to focus on serving, doing, and setting the process in motion to bring comfort and joy to the dying person. It is a commitment I have not regretted.

Chapter Five

The Death

Although a vast mystery surrounds the moment of death and those few days and hours which precede it, the mystery is far less than most of us believe. We know a good deal about that time. Ancient beliefs and traditions inform us, and more recently we have well-documented reports from those who were once "dead" but were then revived. In addition, those in the present hospice movement are acquiring more knowledge, both individually and collectively, about dying. Now, for the first time in many years, we are able to learn directly from people who are dying. What are we being told about the bit of time which surrounds death?

We have learned that there is a time of immediate preparation for death. It begins, generally, about three days prior to the dropping of the dense physical body. Throughout this book I have spoken of the various ways that people cope with illness and the prospect of death; now that work is largely done. The last of one's earthly business is generally resolved, and communication with friends and family decreases or stops altogether. The soul, I believe, takes this time to prepare to leave the body. The person who is dying often knows that death is near; so may attentive observers.

Even in cases of sudden death, there is consistent evidence that the end is subconsciously anticipated. It is not uncommon for surviving relatives to discover that the loved one had recently revised a will, contacted long-lost friends, or settled an old disagreement.

During a protracted death, less medication for pain is needed as death approaches. The body increases the production of endorphin, a morphine-like substance. As the dying person's griefwork is completed, withdrawal becomes more pronounced. Final goodbyes are said, and a stillness ensues. The person's energies, it seems, focus on the spiritual, rather than the physical, plane. The next step is usually a deep sleep or coma. This may be an easy, seemingly normal sleep, or alternatively a restless, tormented half-waking. The variation, I believe, depends on the individual's readiness to die. The person who is still attached to earthly existence struggles; the one who has resolved earthly concerns rests and gathers energy for the next cycle.

Many dying people have made a statement supporting that belief. One woman, near death, but very uneasy, asked her husband, "Do you see those four sets of questions on the ceiling?"

"No, dear, I don't," he said, thinking she was delirious.

"Well, there are four sets of questions on the ceiling," she said firmly. Then her voice took on a worried tone. "I don't know all the answers. I can't leave until I know the answers."

For some time, the woman seemed preoccupied with the questions she saw, although she could not relate either the questions or the answers to others who were near, caring for her. The same woman, somewhat later in her death process, pleaded with a nephew to take off her tight shoes and socks. "They're so tight, they pinch," she said. Her feet were quite bare, of course.

This dying woman's concerns, I believe, were not a result of delirium, but of her clearer consciousness of her situation in the life/death cycle. She clung to life because she literally had not learned all she needed to learn in her lifetime. She longed to be freed from her earthly existence as one longs to take off a shoe that is too tight.

This woman's clarity of language is not unusual among the dying. If we listen, they will tell us about their experiences; too often those close to the dying pass off such descriptions and messages as meaningless hallucinations. As a result, important ideas can be lost.

Within the twenty-four hour period before death, many patients experience what seems to be remarkable improvement. The coma may break, and the dying person is conscious or otherwise cognizant. He or she may speak or smile, ask for one thing or another. For the family, this is an emotionally dangerous period. It seems the hoped-for miracle has happened, that death is averted. This apparent improvement lasts only a short time, however. A rapid decline nearly always follows.

During or before the last twenty-four hours, the body's functions cease; kidney failure is in fact the most frequent direct cause of death. The extremities begin to cool and may take on a bluish color as circulation decreases. Response to sensory stimulation—sound, touch, smell—diminishes. It is my belief that the dying person, however, is able to hear and understand, even after death has apparently occurred. Music, especially then, is appropriate, as is speaking directly to the patient. A caregiver can remind the dying to go toward the light that is perceptable at this time. Remind them to look neither to the right nor to the left of this light, but to go directly toward it. Calm, supportive encouragment, rather than trying to hold them here, is a great comfort to the terminally ill.

As the dying process continues, respiration becomes labored and shallow. The lungs fill with fluid, the dying person's breath bears a liquid sound. Pulse is slower and weaker; blood pressure drops. Sometimes a high fever erupts as the body's temperature control fails. This is the most difficult time for medical personnel to resist emergency treatment or medication. "Couldn't something be given to stabilize blood pressure?" family members ask. "Or to stimulate the heart rate? Could oxygen help the breathing?" It is greatly tempting to relate the fever to a possible infection and consider giving massive doses of an antibiotic, or to devise other tactics to stretch the last bits of life. Other than acting to control the fever symptomatically, however, intervention at this point in the dying process is futile, and only prolongs the dying person's task.

This description of the process of dying is of necessity quite general. Each individual's death is unique, and a given patient may, for instance, undergo a lengthy coma or no coma; may alternate periods of sociability with quiet times; or experience a sudden heart stoppage rather than a gradual slow-down.

In Eastern philosophy, those who are highly evolved find a lovely tree under which they seat themselves, invite their friends to share in the good-bye, and promptly withdraw from the physical body. This is done only when all the work has been completed on this earthly plane.

Since most of us are not yet so evolved, I shall return to what usually happens in the process. As an example of how these elements are combined in an individual case, consider the death of Joann, whose husband of many years, Louis, recorded the changes she experienced.

In mid-November, Joann was diagnosed as having cancer in several organs. Until several weeks after the diagnosis, Joann felt healthy and normal. Her cancer, however, was far advanced. No treatment could help her, so none was attempted. Instead, plenty of pain medication was made available to her, and Louis and Joann visited with friends, traveled a bit, and concentrated on finishing Joann's earthly business. By the first of January, Joann was feeling quite weak. Here is Louis's account of her last few days of life:

January 6—was up several times when I heard Joann getting up to go to the bathroom. Went to bed myself at 8:00 p.m., exhausted. Had one visitor today. Joann is doing a lot of sleeping today—no pain. Had two soft-boiled eggs for breakfast with broth and tea and soup for lunch. After lunch had some jello. Insists upon getting washed and dressed each day. Getting harder and harder as she grows weaker, I manage to snooze during the day until the phone rings. Heard Joann telling today's visitor she is feeling a little stronger today and will probably be showing some improvement. Is still very keen and lucid and interested in mail, etc.

January 7th—Joann ate pretty well today including two glasses of milk and brandy. Keeps her dentures out most of the time since her mouth must be shrinking and the dentures are loose. Her tongue is an ugly brown and cracked and coated. Her skin is very yellow all over, eyes very yellow and feet and legs somewhat swollen.

January 8th—Joann is extremely weak today. She had only orange juice, milk, and cream of farina for breakfast, and a little soup during the day. A friend stopped by with a commode and suggested an egg crate mattress. I obtained one for $15.00.

January 9th—Joann walked to the bathroom and washed, but stayed in her gown. Her breakfast was orange juice and tea; she ate a little soup during the day. One visitor came today.

January 10th—We had quite a few callers, eight in all. Joann seems extremely sleepy but she greeted them all quite cheerfully and knew them by name. She had some soup for lunch with a half glass of wine which she said tasted good. We had some drinks all around and Joann asked for wine but took only a sip. I tried to get her to eat after the callers left, but she only took a sip of milk— saw a great change coming over her; so I decided to make my bed in the living room on the couch and did not undress. About 9:00 p.m. she tried to urinate but I could not raise her out of bed, she was extremely swollen in the body—so much that the marks from the egg-crate pad on her back were very tender to touch. Edema had set in badly. I asked if she wanted to go to the hospital but she said no. I gave her some diapers to urinate in while lying down. Around 11:30 I heard her say, "Now? Now?

Now?" and soon after she called to me to take her to the hospital. I phoned the doctor and he said to get Joann over to the emergency room for a catheter. The ambulance arrived at 12:45 and we were admitted to the Emergency Room at 1:10. The doctor admitted Joann to the hospital. We talked with Joann and she said she was feeling more comfortable. We left her room at 3:00 a.m. and she was very lucid. As we were going out of the house she called from the stretcher to not forget to bring her teeth. So in spite of her discomfort, she had an active mind. Joann waved good-bye after I had kissed her good-night. I returned home much relieved that she was in good hands and that she was not taken to the hospital until she asked for it. I am inclined to think Joann knew her time was near, and she did not want to die at home with me there all alone. I was getting dressed to go to the hospital when the doctor phoned at 10:40 a.m. saying Joann had died peacefully ten minutes earlier. The doctor did not permit any machines but told the nurses to keep her well-sedated. Since Joann had made her own funeral arrangements, all I had to do was call the funeral director and he took over from there.

These changes are indeed frightening in their finality, regardless of one's commitment to a natural, uncomplicated death. But it is important to remember that dying is not an illness to be medicated, excised and cured; it is a process whereby the soul transcends the physical plane for the spiritual one. To accomplish the task, this loved one, the being whom we have grown to love, must shake loose of the body and leave it behind, much as a butterfly, strange and wonderful, leaves its outgrown and useless cocoon.

At last the process is complete. The soul is set free.

In practical terms, what must caregivers do immediately after death? Nothing must be done right away. A quiet, reflective time with the stilled body is useful. There is time to play music, speak of that person's life with others, and consider the meaning of this particular life and death. If the death occurs at home, caregivers and family members may bathe the body, comb the hair, and dress it. All these help reinforce the fact that the life force is gone. If the death is anticipated and arrangements have been made, one need only call the funeral director, when ready, to take the body to the funeral home.

When death occurs in the hospital, the situation requires a different approach. For one thing, medical treatment and monitoring may be a constant interference with the dying process and the emotions of those staying near the dying person. Hospital staff may attempt to restrict "visiting" in the dying person's room or otherwise discourage the presence of loved ones, especially children, although to deny children awareness of the process of dying and death may serve only to reinforce their own fear.

These actions are often well-intended. Often they are simply for the convenience of administration. But family members have the right to keep a vigil with the dying member so long as is necessary. If death occurs while family is not present, it is the family's right to be notified immediately, not after the body has been removed from the room and taken to the funeral home. Viewing the dead body in the hospital bedroom is all part of the grief process, and should always be an available option. When death occurs, it is the family's right to have privacy with the body, rather than being hustled out by staff responsible for preparing the room for someone else.

Death in the hospital need not be impersonal or lonely if caregivers and family assert their rights accordingly. One family gathered to keep vigil at the bedside of their grandmother, an aged woman moving in and out of a deep sleep. Her children and grandchildren took turns looking in on her, speaking softly and recalling family memories. Occasionally a great-grandchild crawled about the floor. At the end of the day, it seemed the grandmother was very near death and the entire family gathered. As the loved ones stood about the grandmother's bed, someone cradled her head, someone else her hand. Soon many arms gently lifted the grandmother and began to rock her. The family began to sing one of her favorite songs: "Rock of Ages, cleft for me, let me hide myself in thee," they sang.

As they rocked the frail body, their grandmother died; yet together the family continued to rock and sing and weep until a great-grandchild's squeal broke the spell. Holding the lifeless body of their grandmother, all looked down to see the smiling, drooling child's face, its chubby hands grasping a toy block which had belonged to the grandmother when she was a child. It was a beautiful and deeply felt moment; all understood at that instant the life and death cycle of constant renewal.

Understanding this cycle is the wisdom which we seek, and which with persistence, we shall find.

Chapter Six

The Funeral

Throughout history people have engaged in rituals and special activities to mark death. Prehistoric Indians in what is now Southern Illinois buried their children with smooth bits of bone tied with tiny beads; in China, rulers were entombed with elaborate ceremony, and sometimes with fully equipped armies skillfully formed of terra cotta. What we do today to mark the end of a loved one's life shares the nature, if not the traditions, of those ancient rites.

Now, as in past centuries, funeral rituals are for the living, for the survivors. We commonly say, "John's funeral" or "the funeral for Edna's mother," when in fact the event is for the survivors. The person who died has gone on to the afterlife and is beyond the sounds of our hymns and eulogies.

It is important to understand the funeral as a societal ritual designed to affirm the sanctity of life—and all our lives—and to confirm the value of that which we give and have been given. I think of a funeral as a gathering of the most important parts of the life that was lived: the dearest people, the most beloved music, the thoughts and ideas that inspired the person who died. Because each life is unique, each funeral should be equally unique. This is why I advocate the prearrangement of funerals by the person who is dying. Caregivers can perform a great service to all involved by opening necessary doors for the dying to accomplish this task.

Prearranging one's own funeral is no longer considered bizarre. Instead, it is now recognized that prearrangement is a considerate gift to the survivors, relieving them of the pressure of decision-making during a time of grief. If the prearrangements are also prepaid, the survivors need not face financial as well as emotional crisis.

Prearrangement also helps the person who is dying. In planning and discussing the funeral, he or she can become more at ease with the impending death by the assurance that the most important aspects of his or her life will be represented in the way that person desires. It also brings a sense of controlling the final ceremony in accordance with beliefs of the deceased. Determining the disposition of the body is often directly related to deeply-held spiritual beliefs. Consequently, it is important for the dying person to be involved, if at all possible, in this decision. I have seen dying made more difficult by anxiety over the question, "What will they do with my body?" When the dying person decides how this question and others will be answered, he or she gains feelings of responsibility, independence, and peace of mind.

By allowing the terminally-ill person to choose and

make basic decisions, prearrangement can also be used to make the funeral a creative expression of life. The personal selection of favorite music and scriptural or other readings can be a source of comfort to the dying person. Listening to recordings of favorite songs and selecting one or more for inclusion in the funeral ceremony is useful. "I want my friends to remember me whenever they hear this song," is a request I have often heard. Another is: "We'll have to play that at the funeral because that's what my life is all about." Some prefer traditional Bible readings, such as the Twenty-third Psalm; others would rather choose contemporary or romantic poetry or a passage from a particular book. Other considerations include the selection of musicians, flowers, and in some cases the design of the ritual itself.

Prearranging the funeral must also involve the funeral director and the immediate survivors as well as clergy, if one is to be included in the ceremony. To a lesser or greater extent, the needs of these individuals must also be accommodated, else it is quite likely that the prearrangements will be altered to suit the survivors.

Family members may feel strongly about the disposition of the body. For instance, the daughter of a woman I worked with confided that she dreaded the cremation of her mother's body. She couldn't stand the thought, she said, because she herself had suffered painful burns as a child. The mother had not realized the depth of her daughter's feelings. Together, they came to an understanding about the cremation after reminiscing about the long-ago accident.

Funeral plans should involve only the immediate family. This is no time for aunts, uncles, or cousins to be consulted, unless a given relationship is extraordinarily close. The group planning the funeral, led by the dying person, should remain as small as possible. Otherwise, conflicting needs and ideas are more likely to impede progress, while exhausting the energy and patience of everyone. The caregiver can aid this delicate process of negotiation and compromise by encouraging open communication. When tempers flare or wills falter, this is a critical and valuable role.

The caregiver can also help with the paperwork from various government and insurance agencies, tasks that are confusing enough during happy times, let alone during bereavement. A caregiver may help survivors understand the various methods of disposing of the loved one's body. Cremation is now widely practiced, and may be an alternative of choice for some families. Many people nonetheless equate cremation with "burning up the body" and focus on visions of terrifying destruction. While cremation is, in fact, burning, it also hastens the natural oxidation process by which all natural matter, embalmed or not, returns to its most basic compounds. Ashes simply become ashes faster. In many areas costly burial plots and containers are not required after cremation; furthermore, some areas allow the ashes to be scattered over particularly beloved places, as the author Joy Adamson's ashes were scattered over the lion country of Kenya. When those planning the funeral fully understand the facts pertaining to cremation, they often feel freer to choose it.

The planners may also be encouraged to understand the work of the embalmer and make decisions affecting its outcome. Some survivors, accustomed to seeing the dying person as pale and fragile-looking, are unpleasantly startled to see the prepared corpse rouged and wigged and dressed up; others may wish to see the body restored to some semblance of health. The caregiver can tactfully assist the planning group to explore their feelings, and communicate with the embalmer accordingly.

Family members should also be made aware of policies governing the donation of bodies for medical research or organ transplants. The group needs to know that they may be asked to pay to transport the body back from the medical facility if it is refused for any of a variety of reasons. If organs are accepted for transplant, the recipients may remain unknown. This knowledge may influence the decisions the group makes.

Others outside the family may be involved in pre-arranging the funeral. These mainly include clergy and funeral directors, but may also extend to representatives of organizations such as the Masons, who may be asked to participate in gravesite rites. When the patient leads the planning, these individuals are usually open to visiting with the group as the dying person's condition allows.

Dealing with the clergy can be comforting or disquieting, depending on the religious orientation of the dying person and surrounding loved ones. Also, individual clergy vary in their ability to cope with the situation. If the caregiver knows the family and the clergyman well, he may be able to aid accordingly. Some ministers are quite flexible and willing to tailor the funeral to the desires of individuals involved; others are rigid, insisting upon the use of church-dictated ritual, allowing only certain Biblical passages to be read, and so on. If a dying person who is planning his or her own funeral meets inordinate resistance from the clergy, the caregiver may remind the person that many funerals are now held in funeral home chapels, and this method is quite acceptable. It is no longer necessary to use churches for funerals; not only clergy now preside at funerals.

Clergy can be very helpful in assisting the dying and survivors understand the church rituals advocated for use during funerals. The funeral rituals of many churches seem cold and selfserving; the element of human comfort which is the genesis of funerals seems buried deep under centuries of repetition of the ritual. The clergy can interpret the meaning of rituals, explaining the Bible readings, and in general, educate the dying person and the family.

The role of the funeral director is also one of educating and serving the family. This person can explain the various formats which can be used for funerals, as well as give information about the treatment of the body immediately after death. While unscrupulous funeral directors are far less common than some believe, it is nonetheless helpful for the care-

giver to become familiar with the state's rules and re-
gulations pertaining to the funeral industry and thus
act as an independent source of information for the
survivors. The funeral director, besides handling the
body after death and providing vehicles for the funeral procession, may also provide a viewing room,
the use of the chapel, and other facilities. The funeral
director may be called upon to read the service as
well. The director is also obligated to disclose the
costs of all materials and services used in connection
with the funeral.

When agreement about the funeral is reached, each
detail should be written out completely and the document signed by all involved. (I am, by the way, per-
sonally in favor of each adult having on file, like a will,
arrangements for his or her own funeral. These should
be updated every few years as needs and perceptions
change. Unfortunantly, signed documents stating intentions and desires for the funeral service do not
have the legal status of wills, but the very act of
signing such a document causes most people to feel
committed to seeing the stated intentions become
reality.)

Should the desires of the dying person not be properly understood and acknowledged, there is a good
chance that details will not be as that person hoped it
would be. In the absence of a clear and lasting expression of intent from the person who has died, the
funeral director will abide by the wishes of the family
members who, in the midst of grief, may also make decisions not in accordance with previous agreements.

Does it matter if the wishes of the dying person get shoved aside in favor of the preference of the living? I believe it matters a great deal, for the funeral ceremony which is prearranged by the dying person is the last earthly expression directly from that person to loved ones. The prearranged funeral is given in trust, so it should be received in equal trust. Also, the grief-work of the survivors is often made more difficult by a change in the funeral arrangements. In the event of sudden death, survivors usually must plan the funeral. A caregiver can be helpful to them as well. The funeral planning must be done quickly, of course, but the caregiver who has the opportunity to help plays essentially the same role.

Many survivors recall few details of the funeral after only a few days. One woman I counseled repeatedly stated that while there had been a gravesite service for her husband, she had not attended it. Upon further questioning, however, she finally said, "Oh, of course I went to the gravesite ceremony. That's how I got the flag—they gave it to me there." This woman had closely tended her ill husband for a long while before he died. There seems to be some correlation between the amount of involvement a survivor had with the dying person and the level of awareness of the proceedings of the funeral, but it is not a strong one. That is, survivors who have anticipated the death of a loved one are not necessarily more serene or aware of funeral proceedings than are others. It may take months of griefwork for a survivor to recall, when hearing a particular melody, that the song was used at the funeral.

For family and close friends, the funeral gives opportunity for one last good-bye. Beyond this, however, the ceremony also serves to create a sense of closure and emphasizes the finality of death. Regardless of the particulars of how the death came about, it is at the funeral that the fact of death is at last acknowledged, spoken about openly, and reinforced.

If a survivor remained at the side of the loved one until the end, the sense of closure may also involve the final laying down of the burden of care. Comfort can be found in no longer needing to keep constant watch over the dying person's condition or witnessing the indignities illness brings. This is not the reaction of a selfish person who rejects difficulty as quickly as possible. Instead, it is the healthy response of an honorable worker who has undertaken a strenuous task and who, when it is completed, is entitled to feel relief and a sense of accomplishment. It is entirely appropriate at the time of the funeral for the survivor to consider new beginnings as well as to review the life of the loved one.

While grief overrides these other feelings, it is healthy for the survivor to experience relief and a sense of freedom at this time. There are, of course, all sorts of emotions and behavior evident at funerals. In my work I've seen families degenerate into warring camps and individuals soaking in private pools of gloom, isolated from those who could—and would—give great solace if allowed. Some stride crisply through a funeral as though attending a business meeting, and others behave in ways that distract others—and themselves—from the funeral proceedings. For instance, at my father's funeral one of his friends oddly persisted in behaving like a clown, popping out from doorways at me, hissing "Boo!" and making silly faces. I was hardly a child at the time and felt genuinely offended. Now I understand that the man, out of his own discomfort and inability to deal with my father's death, was seeking to distract me and, I'm sure, lessen my pain. All I could think at the time was "You fool! My father's dead and you're playing peek-a-boo!" I would have been more compassionate with him now.

There are also those among the deceased's close friends and family who refuse to attend the funeral because they "don't know how to act," "get too upset," or "think funerals are pagan, useless rituals; after all, the dead person is gone.." These excuses are markedly similar to those used by those who cannot seem to bring themselves to visit the dying person. A funeral is, above all, an acknowledgement of mortality, a time in which all reflect upon their own lives and deaths. Those who refuse to attend funerals refuse to allow themselves that reflection; thus they deny their own intimate connection with death and preserve their own false sense of security. Facing death can be scary and requires courage, but not to face it means that life is spent in unreality and death, when it must be faced, will be terrifyingly strange. Those people who deny facing death are doing what is easiest, not what is best for the understanding of their own mortality. From my own experience, most funerals are attended by those to whom the funeral can be an enriching, life-affirming experience, and by those to whom it is just another social obligation.

Funeral rites generally begin with a visitation or viewing, even when the casket remains closed. Visitation is usually the first time the family sees the body after the embalmer has completed the necessary work. Visitation is also a public occasion and places pressure on the family to provide leadership, poise, and good taste to the occasion. These expectations are, of course, unreasonable, but they exist. A caregiver can help the survivors deal with these pressures by assuring them that this is an appropriate time to grieve openly and to take comfort in the company of others who share their feelings. They do not need to be pillars of strength upon which others lean.

The caregiver may also work "behind the scenes" to assure that the family is prepared for the viewing of the body. This can be very important to the survivors. On the day of his wife's funeral, I received a telephone call from Bill, who the day before had asked me the poignant question, "Is it possible to love too much?"

"Elizabeth," he asked hesitantly, "could you meet me at the funeral home? I don't think this is Lorna."

At the funeral home, I saw a body which only vaguely resembled Lorna's. It wore a brunette wig which covered the forehead to the eyebrows. The death pallor was covered by heavy makeup. One button of the dress was unbuttoned, something modest Lorna would never have allowed. The neck was marred by a discoloration.

After ascertaining that the body was indeed Lorna's, I asked the funeral director if I could change a few things. While the family stood nervously among the flowers in the viewing room, I removed the wig, which was held in place by a large pin through the scalp. With a comb and some water, I arranged her wisp gray hair into the pixie style she had worn for as long as I had known her. I fastened the button of the dress to close the gap. The funeral director covered the mark on the neck with make-up.

The family then saw, with relief, the Lorna they had known. "What about her glasses?" someone asked. "She doesn't need them anymore," another family member responded. After some discussion, it was agreed that the glasses would not be used. The funeral went on as planned, but Lorna's family could have been spared this anxiety had they been better informed of the ways in which bodies are usually prepared for viewing.

My thoughts on viewing the body—either during the funeral ceremony or during a separate time—have completely changed from the time of my father's death. I then thought it useless and morbid. Now I believe that actually seeing the dead body helps affirm the fact of death in the minds of viewers. Some, of course, do not deal well with the very real presence of a dead body, but they ought to have the opportunity to face the fact. Further, one's initial response to seeing the body is not all that occurs. A person who seems unable to cope with viewing at the moment often later internalizes the reality and benefits from it.

Because of my belief in the importance of this reality, I do not encourage the body being made up to appear healthy or young again. This veil is not needed. Why are survivors denied the reflection of mortality which is the central purpose of the ritual? But funeral directors defend the beautification of the dead body by stating that the public demands it. This is all part of the conspiracy of death, and we are the perpetrators because of our own needs to continue denying death as an integral part of life.

There is currently some debate between the use of flowers at funerals and donations of money to various charities or memorial funds. This need not be an either/or situation. Memorial contributions are loving gifts which help carry on the work or concern of the person who died. Flowers at a funeral have an entirely different—and equally important—purpose. A contribution is practical, while flowers are symbolic; the two ought not to be compared. Often the family will provide the flower arrangement that covers the casket and then ask friends to make monetary contributions to the deceased's favorite organization. There are hundreds of worthwhile charities that would gratefully accept memorial gifts and this should be a part of the prearranging process.

If musicians are available to play at the funeral, their contributions can add immeasurably to the ceremony. A friend of mine once attended the funeral of a musician who had played with a swing band. His long-time comrades played for his funeral and filled the chapel with upbeat, joyous sounds. Spirits were lifted that day as the remaining members of the band played a jazzy version of "Swing Low,Sweet Chariot" and a darkly melodious and powerful "Rock of Ages." Truly, that funeral was a gathering together of the best parts of the musician's life.

Another funeral is clearly etched in my memory. Sharon Wilson had planned her own funeral, dictating to me over the telephone: "For music, I want someone to sing "My Way," and I want the service to be held at the little stone church. Read the Twenty-Third Psalm. Here's who I want there," and she rattled off many names. "Call them!" she continued. "Don't make it too long, and I want everyone to have a party afterward. And I have this other idea I want done—you'll need about 150 carnations."

Sharon's plans were carried out, and her funeral became a real celebration of life. As people came to the church, school children from her daughter's class handed a single perfect carnation to each—and the 150 flowers were not enough. At the end of the ceremony. led by Sharon's daughters, each person attending filed to the front of the church. Those with carnations placed them in Sharon's favorite copper vase which had been set on the altar. Symbolically, each person had been given a lovely bit of Sharon's life; then, each had returned that gift in equal love. The participants then held hands to form a large, interlocking circle with the bouquet in the center, just as Sharon was in the center of their thoughts. Together, all recited the Twenty-Third Psalm. Finally, the ceremony was adjourned to a party downstairs, as Sharon had requested. It was wonderful—a real celebration of Sharon's life and a true recognition of her value to us.

Sharon chose not to have a gravesite service, as was her right. I think, however, that gravesite services are very important and that our society does not use them in the best possible way. Typically, gravesite services are short. The family and some others gather with the casket and the flowers and the clergy. A few words are said, and perhaps a symbolic handful of earth is thrown into the grave. Anyone who begins to weep loudly is hustled away, and all leave. Then strangers with a crane-like contraption and a bulldozer lower the casket, shove earth into the grave and tramp it down. Flowers are propped over the grave and the job is done.

Gravesite services would be much more useful to survivors if they stayed to watch the lowering of the casket and actually filled the grave, shovelful by shovelful, themselves. The burial is so final and so real that it cannot fail to impress survivors. The reason gravesite services exist as they presently do, I believe, is to shield survivors from the reality of death and to shield others from being disturbed by some becoming emotionally distraught. This "protection" delays an important part of griefwork.

The gravesite services for a young man who died in a motorcycle accident in Georgia were a refreshing contrast to the usual customs. His most important peers were the members of his motorcycle club, and this group, with the cooperation of his parents, planned and carried out his funeral. A lovely picture of his beloved cycle was airbrushed inside the hood of the young man's casket. The body was dressed in fine "show leathers," and placed beside it in the casket were a six-pack of beer, a favorite mug, and several sexy magazines. The motorcycle club members conducted the ceremony, which was held in the funeral home chapel.

The procession to the gravesite was truly impressive. Seventy-five huge motorcycles ridden by stern young men and women dressed in their finest led the way. Even the deceased's black Labrador dog rode in a side car wearing goggles, as it had often ridden with its master. For this funeral procession, unlike others, traffic cleared away as butter from a hot knife.

At the gravesite, the motorcyclists gave a final 16-gun salute to their friend. Then they lowered the casket into the grave and, passing the shovel from hand to willing hand, members filled and mounded the grave. "We looked after him when he was alive," one of the leaders said, his arms around the grieving parents. "We won't abandon him now."

This was a gravesite service that truly allowed the finality of the young man's death to be acknowledged and let the healing among survivors begin. No one who broke into loud weeping was escorted away. Those who became unsteady on their feet were merely helped to sit down safely and continue their griefwork. No signal was given for all to "go home." After a time, a silent consensus was reached and individuals drifted toward their vehicles when they felt the time was right to leave. It was a moving closure to the young man's brief but deeply-shared life.

There is another tradition, held in some regions of the country, which also is very warm and healing. This is the funeral dinner. It is often held at the home of the deceased or at the church and follows the gravesite services. A friend of mine related the dinner which followed her aged grandfather's funeral. All her life he had seemed very old to her, and he had been ill for a very long time. She was startled when the car in which she was riding turned from the cemetery toward the church instead of toward home, as she expected. She was more amazed when told that they would attend the dinner put on by the ladies of the church. "Good grief," she thought. "We just buried Grandpa. Who wants to eat?"

She soon found that eating was not the point of the dinner, although the food was plentiful and good. As plates were filled and conversation began, people a-round her began to speak of her grandfather as they had known him. The young woman learned for the first time of her grandfather's first wife who died after only a few years of marriage, leaving him heartbroken for years (he had always treated girls and women gruffly when she knew him). Tales of his capricious early years were swapped across the table, and she learned of some of the triumphs he had experienced in his life.

To the young woman's amazement, her perception of her grandfather's life enlarged and changed radically. No longer did he seem a sorry old man in failing health and befuddlement at the end of his years. Instead, in her mind she saw the variety of his life in its long span, including the love and grief he had felt, struggles he had endured, and gains he had made. "I came away refreshed," she said. "All those people together gave me a sense of my heritage from Grandpa and the courage to live my life as well as he did. My grief over his death ebbed away and was replaced by a desire to carry on in his traditions."

Shared strength and comfort is the main course of the funeral dinner which is designed to nourish the grieving soul as well as the body.

One more concern. Throughout too many modern funeral ceremonies, from the viewing to the gravesite service, there is a tendency to isolate those who give themselves over to grief. Sobbers are hushed and wailers escorted out. Tranquilizers of various sorts are often pressed upon those who grieve loudly or openly. In truth, these people who give full rein to their bereavement are doing what is right and healthy for them, and others should respect their way instead of diverting or stifling them. It is my observation that those who react physically, emotionally, and verbally to their grief are usually reaching the climax of their griefwork and will soon begin to resolve their hurt. To deny the full expression of grief is to delay healing.

When the final bouquet of life is gathered and each bloom examined and shared, survivors may go forward with their lives, feeling that the closure to the loved one's life was right and good. The funeral, then, is a precious, final gift in honor and affirmation of that life lived—and also of ours.

Chapter Seven

Survivors

From the hour I heard of my father's death until I entered therapy years later, I was a wretched example of a survivor who had not done her griefwork. When my sister called to tell me, I screamed denials, cursed God, wept bitterly. For years I could not say Dad's name without tears, nor tolerate even the mildest criticism of him. My grief was a great burden which threatened to crush me. I struggled mightily against grief, as I struggled against all other "bad" things and feelings in my life.

Several events contributed to my inability to cope with my grief. First, the funeral had to be rescheduled. Ironically, Dad had always made it a point to arrive a few minutes late for any family or business meeting. This habit annoyed my mother, a punctual woman who would grit her teeth and admonish: "Henry, you'll be late for your own funeral!" And true to form, as the town merchants prepared to close their shops in honor of a respected neighbor, the arrangements finalized and the family members gathered, word came that Dad would be late. The plane carrying his body was fogged in at a German airport; a 24-

hour delay was necessary.

The dark humor of this situation escaped me at the time. The delay only meant another day of agony for me, another day without fully knowing in my heart if what they said was true, that Dad was dead. While others relaxed somewhat and began to enjoy each other's company, I held myself,tight—and apart from everyone.

When Dad's body arrived, it was necessary that someone from the family formally identify it. My husband quickly offered to attend to this awful task. The family custom had always been to protect the women and the young from unpleasantness. When I asked to go along, I was told, "No, you wouldn't recognize him anyway. His body has become very swollen."

If only I could have seen even Dad's hand as his body lay in the casket! I would have recognized at least the shape of his fingers, the size of his fingernails, the sprigs of hair between his knuckles. But throughout the whole confusing day, I was diverted one way or another from facing the reality of Dad's death. I remember standing in the driveway of the funeral home staring at the garage from which the hearse would soon roll, thinking, "This is just a bad dream, and soon I will wake up."

Waking up took five painful years for me. My unresolved grief adversely affected my life and relationships. Since then I have come to a new understanding of his death.

When I last saw Dad, we were at one of those orange-roofed restaurants that line our highways, and

Mom had not yet decided about traveling with him to Germany on the business trip. He persistently urged her to go, and made it clear that his request was very important to him.

Mother did finally make the trip, and while in Germany, they decided to visit Dusseldorf, his birthplace. Dad suffered a massive heart attack. He died quickly, in Mother's arms.

Now I believe that Dad, consciously or not, suspected the end was near, and did his best to arrange his death the way he wanted it to be. Given that we all must die, would we not prefer to die without great ado, in a place we love, and in the arms of a beloved and loving person? My father died this way; his death was good for him because he was able to choose his own surroundings. It is clear to me now that my reactions to his death were based on my feelings of insecurity, my need for my father, my "attachment" to his presence in my life. Had I thought with real love about Dad—*his* life, *his* situation, *his* death—my griefwork could have been accomplished more easily, and I would have been a healthier person.

My experience is not unusual. I needed help in coping with the reality of Dad's death. I needed to resolve my feelings of rejection and anger, and I needed to try to see the event from a perspective other than my own. To meet similar needs is my current goal as I help survivors deal with death. In fact, survivors often require more of my energy than do the dying.

Survivors' emotions are varied and strong. Depression, guilt and frustration abound. Suicidal wishes or statements are not uncommon. Some survivors pray for their own illness or death. Frequently anger predominates, often directed at the medical team or others who were believed to be "in charge." But I have also seen families come into the doctor's office the day after the death to thank the medical team for its efforts.

Regardless of the surrounding circumstances, grief-work must be done—and the process is correctly called "work." It's hard; it's sometimes long. Occasionally it seems so difficult that the worker may never get it done. Each individual brings to the situation his or her own personal experiences, abilities and ideas, and responds to grief accordingly.

If the survivor was obsessively attached to the person who died, he or she may be entirely overcome with guilt and the pain of separation. Seeing survivors in this situation reminds me of a lovely presision-made shiny cap I once had on one of my molars. It was a beautiful, smooth thing that covered an unsightly damaged tooth, and it slipped off its perch during a cocktail party. Beneath it, to my surprise, the real tooth was rotting, coming loose with decay.

How like our lives. We spend so much energy with the outward things—our appearance, our belongings, our social amenities—covering up the real aspects of the relationship. We go along trying to ignore the anger, guilt, resentment, and other unresolved emotions within a relationship. When it comes to its final end, as happens in death, the survivor will sooner or later be stricken with the reality of needing to resolve them. Unless those feelings are resolved, the survivor may become unable to continue with a healthy and productive life, for the decay will not be cleansed any other way. When the task is accomplished, the survivor can learn from the relationship that was, and from the ending of it. Certainly the death of one close to us causes loneliness and emptiness. These feelings and others which might accompany them, however, need not shut off the potential to learn positive lessons from the relationship. At first these emotions are all mixed up and jumbled; it takes time to sort out feelings and relationships.

In working with survivors, I focus on thoughts of love and compassion. I answer their questions, both medical and otherwise, and seek out the answers to questions I can't answer right away.

One ritual that I've found to be very helpful to survivors is the disposal of medications, especially if the dying person was cared for in the home. There usually is an array of accumulated bottles and boxes and tubes and trays of this and that. We take each one, look at it, and read the name of the medication. From there, I guide the conversation to the infirmity which that particular drug was to have countered. For instance, the morphine is no longer necessary because there is no more pain; the Lasix rids the body of excess fluids, and that's no longer necessary. And so on we go until we've discussed each prescribed drug.

This opens the door for the survivor to recall the depredations of the illness and for the counselor to reinforce the concept of the necessity of death, the relief from discomfort, and the quality of the efforts of the medical team. It also allows both to emphasize that the struggle is over. As each medication is dropped into the disposal box, a little pain and grief goes with it, until all the medication has been taken away. Usually the survivor gives a great sigh of relief to see the stuff gone, and takes a giant mental step away from overwhelming grief.

Later, the survivor may want to discuss spiritual beliefs related to death. Sometimes it is important only for the survivor to reiterate his or her beliefs, aloud and uninterrupted. The counselor need only nod or give other quiet encouragement. After the "work" is completed for such a session, I give the survivor a hug and let him know of my support. Often touching or holding while this "work" is being done disrupts the trend of thought and the person may stop sharing.

Occasionally survivors want more discussion, and a counselor must use his or her best judgement in expressing personal spiritual beliefs. I believe strongly, for instance, in life after death and embrace the concept of rebirth; otherwise, for me death would be the absolute end of a beloved being and thus something to struggle against and to hate. But I do not always discuss these beliefs with survivors, particularly those whose own beliefs are in opposition to mine and might use my beliefs as a focus for misdirected anger. To offer my beliefs inappropriately might only serve to anger, confuse, or depress a survivor; so while I am not reluctant to share my beliefs, I do so only when it is responsible and genuinely helpful to the survivor. Strong spiritual beliefs, regardless of denomination, can carry a survivor through periods of grief. Alice, a woman I worked with, was the main caregiver of her dear friend Anna. The two shared a friendship Alice described as "awe-inspiring" and an abiding faith in God which strengthened them both. Alice wrote this account of their struggle together:

It seems like Anna was sick for a very long time, yet as I look back it went so quickly. In October, 1974, Anna was hospitalized. After several tests, one of which was the terrifying pneumo-encephalogram, she was discharged without being told the results. She was to learn later that her physician suspected a degeneration or demylenization of the central nervous system, or multiple sclerosis. Anna was not aware of this until the diagnosis was confirmed in April, 1978. After many tears and prayers, we started searching for hope and treatment. Thank you, God, for her determination.

Anna spent long, agonizing hours doing her theraputic exercises. She spent two weeks at the rehabilitation clinic three different times. Thank you, God, for her courage.

By January, 1979, Anna was using a quad cane to help her balance. In April, this was replaced by a walker. At that time, Anna said, "The next step is a wheelchair," and she was right. We kept on exercising and praying, praying and exercising. We prayed constantly for a miracle. We knew that it would have to be a miracle to halt the progression of the disease. Then came the wheelchair and the day that Anna could no longer attend her beloved church. We shed many tears because of this but did not give up. Anna trusted God. She said that He knew what He was doing—who were we to question? Thank you, God, for her trust.

July 15, 1979, is a day that will be stamped indelibly in my memory. The doctors had rediagnosed Anna's illness as ALS, amyotrophic lateral sclerosis. We had never heard of this, and it was frightening. I had taken Anna for treatments three consecutive Fridays in May. At last, the neurologist who gave her these treatments dealt me a rough blow. He had Anna taken from the room and explained to me the nature of this horrifying disease. He also told me that her life would be over in a matter of months.

To say I was shattered is putting it mildly. I offered up a quick prayer for courage and a plea for strength and asked forgiveness in advance for the deceit that I was going to live for a while. I could not tell Anna—I had to face her and drive her home, making idle chatter while my heart was breaking and my head was pounding with the new knowledge that my beloved friend had a terminal illness. Thank you, God, for Anna's faith.

From that time on, we lived under the shadow of death. We prayed like we never prayed before. We filled our days talking about many different things. We drew closer together and closer to God. I think that this is when I started to mourn. I could see the change in Anna day by day. She could no longer exercise. With each stage I experienced more and more grief. I couldn't bear the thought of life without Anna, nor could I bear the heartache of watching her lose so much so quickly. First her balance, then her walking, then her coordination, her sitting up, the use of her arms. Her mind remained sharp and clear. She was always one step ahead of me. She remained strong in her beliefs. Thank you, God, for her strength.

Thanksgiving was the last meal that Anna managed to come to the dinner table for. After that, I fed her in her room. Her courage and fortitude were an inspiration to all of us. She touched so many lives, she would not give up. She had tremendous will to live, so great that she defied medical science by living as long as she did. Thank you, God, for her courage.

Anna never lost her sense of humor. No

matter how much pain she had, she always had a smile. Thank you, God, for her beauty.

On Wednesday, May 20, 1980, God called my beloved friend home. She died as she lived, quietly and trusting in her Lord. Part of me died with her just as part of her lives with me.

Thank you, God, for her life. Anna is with her beloved Savior now. Walking with Jesus. Her legacies are an undying faith in God, her wit and wisdom and her love for all people. She is at peace, but I am not. I am still struggling with my selfish grief. My sorrow and loss are overwhelming. I pray that God will grant me the Grace to fill my emptiness and the strength to bear the hurt. He gave us a promise, Revelation 7:17: "And God shall wipe away all tears from their eyes." The Will of God will never lead you where the Grace of God cannot keep you.

Anna believed this—so must I. The force of yesterday's tears is not as strong as the love of God which gives us the strength to start a new day. Through my sad loss others may see the lesson in faith as I carry on in God's name. I shall not charge these heart-aches to Him—He is perfect love and real love does not hurt us. He is standing by more tenderly than ever to help and He is the only one who can put the sunshine back in my heart. Thank you, God, for Anna.

Alice, though deeply grieved by Anna's death, held within her the resolution to go forward in life. Having fought side-by-side with Anna, she had focused her anger on the illness itself, not on other people.

Not all survivors cope with death in this manner. My friend Louise was not a bit subtle about her feelings at the death of her husband, John. They had been married for more than forty years and their lives were deeply intertwined.

I went to visit her two weeks after John's death. We had often talked about the possibility of John dying. Louise was sitting on a lawn chair, wearing a faded, pink quilted robe with a pink knitted shawl around her shoulders. She had lost twenty-two pounds and seemed vulnerable.

"Oh, Louise," I said, "You look so sad, as if you'd like to die, too."

"Oh, God, yes," she responded. "If there is a God, every night I go to bed and pray that He will stop my heart from beating." Louise's sorrow was in her face and her voice.

"And then what?" I asked.

Without a moment's hesitation, she snapped, "I will find John no matter where he is, and when I do, I'll kiss him all over his body, and then I'll kick his rear end for leaving me!"

Louise's feelings were pure and direct. She was angry, and she was angry at John. At 70, Louise resolved her grief finally, by deciding to carry on her life as though John was on an extended trip to a destination far away. While he was out of her sight, then he was not out of her mind (at least not for long, ever); she spoke of John as if she would be seeing him after his long journey. She went on the same as before, anticipating meeting John again.

Most widows and widowers must make far greater adjustments. An incredible amount of letting go must occur. The husband of one attractive young woman died after an illness of only six days. By the time she realized he was seriously ill, he was dying. By the time that fact had sunk in, he was dead, and she was left with dizzying confusion and grief.

Her griefwork was long and hard, but she began letting go of her husband and their life together with courage. To her dismay, she soon found that she also had let go of her husband's doctor, who had given her emotional support through the ordeal, and then let go of many of her friends who found it "awkward" to include a single woman in their activities.

As the young woman struggled to understand and cope with the many drastic and unexpected changes in her life, she realized that a crisis was approaching. The first holiday without her husband was Father's Day. What would she do? What would be best for her children? She decided to do as the family had always done: have a cookout.

Cheerfully the young widow began to recreate the annual tradition. She planned the menu and made the grocery list. She decided which child would do what chore. Maybe it was when she was thinking of who would cook, or how many steaks to buy, or whether or not to get the special kind of expensive pickles, but somewhere in the process the plain fact occurred to the young woman that her husband was dead. Gone. Not to return. Their life together was over, and their holiday cookouts with special pickles were over. The central figure that had lent such a glow to that previous life was gone. The vague reality with which she had struggled so long became clear to her, and to her surprise, it didn't hurt.

She began again to plan for the holiday, and as a result, she and her children went on an extended trip to Canada. They went with some sorrow and trepidation, occasionally thinking, "I wish he were here to en joy this." But all returned having made a significant break with the past and feeling a greater sense of completion within themselves. For the young woman and her children, it was the beginning of the end of their griefwork.

I have observed that survivors who have a great deal of difficulty letting go suffer greater anguish during their mourning period. They become more frequently and more deeply depressed, and stay depressed longer than do others who let go more easily. A wise counselor or caregiver can help a deeply grieving survivor most by making frequent contact by phone, mail, or in person, and repeating in any variety the basic and most needed message: "I love you, I will be here for you." Some survivors must simply walk that dark and lonely path of grief alone, but a caregiver may also trail close behind.

Survivors who stayed close to the loved one during the death generally have a shorter period of griefwork than others, but it may be no less intense. The mourning usually begins before death occurs, but survivors still experience shock and disbelief. Jane, Bill's wife, found the grief process dreadfully painful although she'd been by her husband's side throughout his illness and had shared support and comfort with him right to the end. Two days after Bill died, she told me she saw an apparition of her husband standing in the bathroom, tall and whole as he once was.

"I screamed," she said. "I thought I was going crazy. But he—it—Bill—just stood there until my son got up the stairs to my side. Then he disappeared."

"Jane," I said, "do you think that might have been Bill's way of letting you know he's okay, that you can go on now? He was sick and weak for a long time, and you saw him well and strong. I believe in those kinds of messages."

There comes a time in the griefwork when the survivor is ready to sort out the facts of the relationship. This point comes earlier or later; for me, it came when my therapist suggested I write down, as a bit of "homework," some of the things I hadn't liked about my father. Hadn't she heard me say over and over how I loved him, missed him, wanted him back, I thought. Where had she gotten the idea I didn't like Dad, and what in the world would I write?

I put my doubts aside, however, and began to plan my assignment; after all, the therapist was an expert and costing me plenty. If I was to write out some things about Dad, I would have to reach for every one of my memories of him, and examine each one, turning it over in my mind and remembering the details. So I began, and as one does when sorting out one's attic, I went first to those well-loved things; memories of Dad's smile, his honors and accomplishments, and his special way of gently teasing me. As I progressed through my assortment, however, I came upon some memories I had forgotten. And then, as I reached into the dark far corners of my mind, I found some memories I didn't know had been stored there. I also realized that I didn't need all those memories and thoughts, and that I had devoted a good deal of mental energy—not to mention five years of my life—to maintaining them.

So I decided to hold a mental "garage sale." I categorized my memories as ones I wanted to keep— those best loved—and I expanded that group a bit from the store of things I'd forgotten. And then I took pencil in hand and began to list those memories, feelings, and thoughts that were unpleasant in some way: confusing, frustrating or simply unimportant. I would let these go, not hold them or keep them anymore.

Here are some of the things on my "garage sale" list:

- As a child, I hated polishing Dad's shoes every day.
- I felt insulted that he paid me a quarter a week to polish his shoes.
- I didn't like my forced job at Dad's office; riding into New York City on the trains, ferry boat and subways, working at a switchboard, and receiving his wrath if I

accidentally disconnected him from a customer.

- I resented the Sunday duets of my playing the piano while Dad played the violin. He substituted this for really playing with me, claiming he was too busy.
- I resented his not having time enough to be with me, even on weekends, and his "love affair" with the telephone caused painful confrontations between us.

My "garage sale" list eventually filled a page and a half of legal paper. Like used merchandise on a table, my unwanted memories lay displayed there, some acknowledged for the first time. Some were shabby, I knew; and some were unimportant, but most had simply outlived their usefulness to me. I didn't need them anymore. I let them go from my consciousness, and shortly thereafter I was able to begin a fresh new direction in my life.

As a result of my "garage sale," I gained insight into the process of survivors' healing. In acknowledging the range of my feelings toward Dad—resentment, respect, anger and love—I regained a sense of wholeness of our relationship as it had been when he was alive. In the process, Dad lost his god-like place in my memory and once again became the real, complete human being I had known. And I was released to be a real, complete human being, too, as I had been then.

The "garage sale" concept is an important one for survivors. I have used it many times to help survivors sort out and evaluate their feelings and memories, and to use the process as a first step toward getting on with their lives.

What is the resolution of grief? Each person must resolve it in his or her own way, and sort and keep and discard feelings and memories as they will. But the final resolution must be based on love. This seems contrary, for if one had not loved, one would not feel pain in the loss of the loved one. Or at least, wouldn't one hurt less if he'd loved less? Why must love be traded for pain? Bill, Lorna's husband, was turning this thought over in his mind when he asked me after her funeral, if it were possible to "love too much." His response to grief was so painful that his skin was cool and damp and he'd not been able to find his own pulse. His suffering was agonizing.

I had to think about my reply. "No, of course not," was not good enough, although it was true. Eventually, I was able to reply that there are only two ways to avoid grief. The first was to die young, before anyone you love dies. The second is to pass through this life without ever loving anyone.

I have worked with people who have made the second choice and refused to give love, or take it, or be dependent in any way on other people. It is true that they do not suffer the pain or grief at the death of another; what they avoid in life, however, comes to them magnified during death. These people, faced with the end of life, struggle with their last moments, filled with regret and reaping the rejection once sowed. No one escapes the fact of their own humanity; a whole lifetime of denying it does not change it. In my observation, this pain is far greater than the pain of grief; I believe it follows the soul, marking the cosmic consciousness. It is far better to love with all the love within you, without being attached to that person or what he may have to do in life and death.

Unlimited love, however, means an unlimited fullness of life. Loving unconditionally, completely, without strings attached, is the purest form of love. Through our love of others we grow, teach, and learn. In this give-and-take of love, we become more whole and gain something of the essence of the beloved, which we keep forever. This truth makes the pain of grief temporary.

No, Bill, you can't love too much. As you will learn, the joy of having loved lasts forever.

Chapter Eight

Conclusion:

Birthing and Dying

As preparation for birth makes birthing easier, so preparation for death makes dying easier. When a woman goes into labor, she releases all false sense of modesty and attachment to her body, and opens her consciousness to the unknown experiences of birth. Perhaps because of this experience, women who have experienced the birth phenomenon often come to the end of the life cycle with greater acceptance, if not willingness; a greater sureness in releasing themselves once again into the realm of the unknown.

During my previous experience as an obstetrical nurse, I helped with hundreds of births. Now, in my career as a counselor for the dying, I've eased the way for at least that many deaths, and thought often of the question Florida Scott Maxwell once asked: "Is life a pregnancy? That would make death a birth."

Are we who seek to understand the power beyond our earthly existence similar to the unborn child, confined but growing in a darkness which prevents our knowing fully the things we sense? Perhaps our mighty efforts are as the turnings and stretchings of the unborn child, and our lives of seeking understanding a necessary gestation which preceeds a greater destiny. To reach that greater experience, the fetus must be born. And for us to come to know these spiritual forces we now feel—our passage, our transition—is to die.

Birthing compels the child through a dark, narrow passage toward bright light. Those who have survived "clinical death" consistently report a journey through a dark "tunnel" toward a light. As the newborn is received by helping, loving hands, the spirit of the newly-dead is received and advised by the spirits of loved ones who died earlier. When the umbilical cord is cut, the child becomes a self-contained individual, no longer needing direct sustenance from the mother. When death occurs, another, unseen cord is cut and the spirit becomes independent of earthly needs and proclivities. The child begins to learn and grow; the spirit, too, realizes the object of the quest for understanding.

During the last twenty-five years, much has been learned about both birth and death. When my children were born, women were poorly informed about their pregnancies, and little prepared for childbirth. The ideal obstetrical patient took her vitamins and watched her weight, but did not "worry her little head" about the details of the changes she experienced, nor what the future might hold for her. At the onset of labor, women were expected to accept, if not demand, anesthesia. My own birthing experiences,

which were fairly typical, were painful, somew
frightening, and often lonely.

How different things are today! Women are prepared for the birthing process from the time they
choose to conceive.

The most significant shift of focus, however, is toward birth as a family event. When my children were
born, my ex-husband stood aside in some awe and
wonderment—and he is a physician. Today, many
husbands are active participants in childbirth, and
the circle of friends and other relatives (especially
siblings) who may be present at birth is widening. Because couples have demanded freedom from unne-
cessary medical interference, choices like midwifery,
birthing rooms, and birthing chairs are available for
women in labor. Fewer women request anesthesia;
even women who deliver by Caesarian section may remain fully conscious. The birthing of a child today is a
joyous, shared occasion.

Almost simultaneously, another taboo, the discussion of death and dying, began to crumble. The basic
question was this: if everyone who ever lived eventually died, why didn't anyone talk about it? Death,
after all, is more universal than sex. So why didn't
anyone seem to know about death?

The easiest answer, of course, was that no one had
survived death to tell the tale.

However, physicians Elisabeth Kübler-Ross and
Raymond Moody, among others, have reported re-
spectable research on the phenomenon of "clinical
death," which helped change care of the dying from a

purely medical, or physical, problem. Their reports were well-received and widely read. When they were first published, custom dictated that a dying person be hospitalized, often in the most distant wings of the building. Isolated from all but closest family members and subjected to continued and often unwanted treatments, the dying person seemed to take a back seat to the disease which ravaged the body. The medical profession, dedicated to restoring good health, was seldom a source of information about what one could expect while dying. Nurses and doctors saw a patient's death as "losing a struggle" and refused to anticipate the possibility, much less discuss, dying on a personal basis with a patient. To choose to die, to stop treatments, and to try to enjoy the remaining days of life was not a patient's option.

After comparing Kübler-Ross's and Moody's reports with previous notions about death, many people began to confront their beliefs and fears head-on by reading about different aspects of death, attending seminars and discussion groups, and seeking to spend time with the dying.

Many within the medical profession have also listened more closely to the dying. As a result, confinement and isolation of the terminally ill is less common. Patients are no longer expected to accept unwanted procedures which artificially prolong life. Home care is available in many communities, and "hospice" is no longer a strange word. The most important shift of focus, however, is toward death as a shared experience among loved ones, a time when a family may wind a path through pain, fear and grief to resolution, closure, and a joyous affirmation of life. In such cases, one comes to understand the possibility that birth is not the beginning, nor death the end of the life cycle. This life we know is only a middle segment, in which the physical body is donned, then shed. We assume the use of it, keep it for a while, and leave it when we have used it enough. Likewise, the soul exists before birth and lives on after death; the true life cycle is greater than we know. When we truly accept the fact that birth and death are but coefficients of the single process of Life, then we know that we are going through an experience with which our subconscious is already familiar. All of us must be born. In being born, we experience dying. It is just a matter of acknowledging, accepting and activating a similar experience in its two-fold aspect. In each case, we leave one realm of familiarity, and forge our way into another realm or form of Life.

Birth and death are words, semantics. It is Life that is Eternal and forever the same. Life remains Life, both in birth and in the death experience. Each of us may find this out as we enter the different realms of Life, both in the here and the hereafter.

Because we are able to think and act in greater accordance with this new awareness, the dying and their caregivers and families need not be overwhelmed by tragedy nor isolated in their grief and difficulty. The loss of a loved one need not be seen as final and forever. Instead, all involved can help and be helped to not only endure the occurrence of death, but to grow, learn, and become greater spiritually as a result of the experience.

Human worth and dignity can be heightened and affirmed during illness and death; indeed, this is the greatest need of the dying person. As that person prepares to leave this physical plane, he needs to be assured that his life is valued and appreciated, and a source of joy to others. When we as caregivers look closely and thoughtfully upon the situation of one who is dying, we find within our hearts the ability to communicate that joy, that affirmation, that compassion which we feel. Our resulting actions are best when simplest: the gentle touch, the soothing voice, the easy errands and honest respect are the greatest gifts we can give.

We as caregivers can comfort and overcome the three great fears of dying: of pain, of abandonment, and of helplessess. The solutions to these problems are not so complex as we might imagine, and, in fact, spring from the recognition that a dying person is entitled to richness of life, to choices, to associations with loved ones, and, conversely, independence in which to prepare for death.

When these basic human privileges are accorded the dying, all involved attain a sense of dignity; when several people work together for the benefit of the most frail among them, the best of human character surfaces. We are enriched by the experience; if ever humans can be genuinely noble, it is then.

By working with and for the dying, we learn a good deal about ourselves and about others. We see in death something common which lies, one way or another, before each of us; we see in the unique the commonality.

In the process, we can confront and let go of our fears and prejudices. We can overcome our all-too-human tendency to love only those who are compliant, cheerful, and unalterably pleasing to us. We can participate in a greater breadth of human experience than has been accorded us thus far in our lives and devine some part of the path which lies before us. This is a freeing experience which enables us to live to greater depth and with greater feeling than we may have thought possible.

By serving the dying, we can examine death and unravel its mysteries until we no longer fear it. Living continues despite illness and infirmity; living in those circumstances has a special poignance and quality all its own. We can feel the reality of giving love which overcomes difficulty and sorrow. We can *receive* love, too—a love which evolves not from convenient, pleasant circumstances, but one which springs unhindered from the deepest human spirit.

Above all, we can achieve a new hope. Rather than experiencing despair at the inevitability of physical death, we can be uplifted by the hope of an easy conscious death for our loved one. We can share this hope with others surrounding the dying person and thus be instrumental in their comfort and growth.

All these goals are possible. With effort, with conscientious attention to the real needs of the dying person and the survivors, they are indeed probable. Each of us has great potential to achieve these goals, simply because we are capable of love and caring.

Achieving a sense of comfort with death and those who are dying is a complex task, but it is much easier than one might believe. Almost everyone endeavoring consciously to learn about death must sort through many emotions, reexamine and reinterpret previous experiences according to new information, and chart a new path to be navigated with the instruments of unconditional love and an affirmation of life.

My own feelings of peacefulness have come to me because I have given up struggling against life as it is, stopped fighting for the way I *thought* things should be, and stopped seeking experiences I believed should be mine. Instead, I've allowed myself to become a leaf in the brook of life, following its natural currents and pausing over deep pools, but always continuing toward an unseen and larger destination.

Elizabeth S. Callari, R.N., is the Founder and Executive Director of the Center for Awakening, a nonprofit organization that provides care and support services for the terminally ill. Previously she has been Director of Nursing Service of the Elisabeth Kübler-Ross Hospice in Pinellas County, Florida, and has served as Chairperson of the Upjohn Homemakers Advisory Board, as well as a practicing chemotherapy nurse.

Ms. Callari lectures widely to professional and civic groups.

DO YOU HAVE A FRIEND OR RELATIVE WHO
WOULD ENJOY THIS BOOK?
Use the convenient order form below.

Order Form

A GENTLE DEATH: Personal Care giving to the Terminally Ill

YES, please send _____ copies at $7.95 each _____

SUBTOTAL

Tax

Tax: (North Carolina only): 5%   Postage & Handling _____
($1.50 first book
.50 each additional book)

TOTAL _____

NAME _____

ADDRESS _____

_____ Zip _____

Send to: **Tudor Publishers, Inc.**
P.O. Box 3443
Greensboro, NC 27402

Prices subject to change without notice.
Allow 4-6 weeks for delivery.

Our Guarantee: *You must be completely satisfied or return the*
book(s) in undamaged condition within 30
days for a full refund.